Welcome to

THE
EVERYTHING

HEALTH GUIDES

W**hen you're faced** with a pressing health issue, your first instinct is to find out as much about it as you can. With so much conflicting information out there, where can you turn for professional, supportive advice?

Packed with the most recent, up-to-date data, THE EVERYTHING® HEALTH GUIDES help ensure that you get a good diagnosis, choose the best doctor, and find the right medical treatment. With this one comprehensive resource, you and your family members have all the information you could possibly need—at your fingertips.

THE EVERYTHING® HEALTH GUIDES are an extension of the best-selling Everything® series in the health category, which also includes *The Everything® Diabetes Book* and *The Everything® Low Cholesterol Book*. Accessible and easy to read, THE EVERYTHING® HEALTH GUIDES provide specific details and clear examples that relate to your given medical situation. If you're looking for one-stop, all-inclusive guides that allow you to understand and become more in tune with your body, this groundbreaking series is the perfect tool for you.

Visit the entire Everything® series at *www.everything.com*

THE EVERYTHING

HEALTH GUIDE TO

MENOPAUSE

Dear Reader,

Welcome to *The Everything® Health Guide to Menopause, 2nd Edition!* We are happy to offer you this update on a women's health topic near and dear to our hearts. As clinicians, we understand the struggle and confusion that women can experience as they go through menopause, and the importance of having good information for making healthy decisions. As women, we are destined to join our patients in this life-altering phase, and don't think for a moment we don't appreciate how hard it is to make those good decisions in the midst of work, families, and the general chaos that is life.

We hope that this book gives you more than just good information. We hope it also gives you support for this transition as well as permission to explore whatever choices will make menopause comfortable and empowering. We invite you to read it in whatever way suits you—every word just as it was written, only the bits that interest you, or with a glass of wine and your women friends. If it piques your curiosity, answers your questions, or just gives you the language to talk to your doc, we'll feel our mission is accomplished. Onward!

Kate Bracy Kalb and
Kathryn Arendt, M.D.

THE

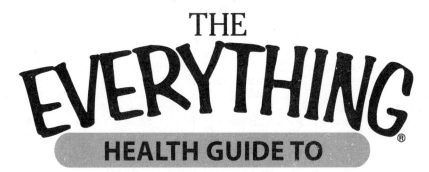

HEALTH GUIDE TO

MENOPAUSE
2nd Edition

Reassuring advice and up-to-date
information to keep you healthy and happy

Kate Bracy Kalb, R.N., M.S., A.R.N.P.

Technical Review by Kathryn Arendt, M.D.

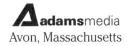
Avon, Massachusetts

This book is dedicated to menopausal women and their partners;
and to Anne, who well knows why.

• • •

Publisher: Gary M. Krebs
Editorial Director: Laura M. Daly
Executive Editor, Series Books: Brielle K. Matson
Associate Copy Chief: Sheila Zwiebel
Acquisitions Editor: Kerry Smith
Development Editor: Brett Palana-Shanahan
Production Editor: Casey Ebert
Technical Reviewer: Kathryn Arendt, M.D.

Director of Manufacturing: Susan Beale
Production Project Manager:
Michelle Roy Kelly
Prepress: Erick DaCosta, Matt LeBlanc
Interior Layout: Heather Barrett,
Brewster Brownville, Colleen Cunningham,
Jennifer Oliveira

An Everything® Series Book.
Everything® and everything.com® are registered trademarks of F+W Publications, Inc.

Published by Adams Media, an F+W Publications Company
57 Littlefield Street, Avon, MA 02322 U.S.A.
www.adamsmedia.com

ISBN 10: 1-59869-405-7
ISBN 13: 978-1-59869-405-5

Printed in Canada.

J   I   H   G   F   E   D   C   B   A

Library of Congress Cataloging-in-Publication Data

Kalb, Kate Bracy.
The everything health guide to menopause / Kate Bracy Kalb. -- 2nd ed.
p.   cm.
"An Everything series book."
ISBN-13: 978-1-59869-405-5 (pbk.)
ISBN-10: 1-59869-405-7 (pbk.)
1. Menopause--Popular works. I. Title.
RG186.K35 2007
618.1'75--dc22
2007018983

This publication is designed to provide accurate and authoritative information with regard to the subject matter covered. It is sold with the understanding that the publisher is not engaged in rendering legal, accounting, or other professional advice. If legal advice or other expert assistance is required, the services of a competent professional person should be sought.
—From a *Declaration of Principles* jointly adopted by a Committee of the American Bar Association and a Committee of Publishers and Associations

Many of the designations used by manufacturers and sellers to distinguish their products are claimed as trademarks. Where those designations appear in this book and Adams Media was aware of a trademark claim, the designations have been printed with initial capital letters.

This book is available at quantity discounts for bulk purchases.
For information, please call 1-800-289-0963.

All the examples and dialogues used in this book are fictional and have
been created by the author to illustrate medical situations.

Acknowledgments

I am very grateful for the opportunity to work on this book. Thanks to Andrea Hurst, my agent, who made the first connection, and to Kerry Smith, my editor, whose patience and instruction were lifesaving. Thanks to all my friends and colleagues who offered ideas about what information should be included, and who helped me keep my perspective through my own menopausal moments. In particular, thanks to my Minnesota writing buddies: Kris, Altha, and Jean. And an enormous thank-you to my family, who tiptoed around weekend after weekend and never once asked me to find their car keys or do the dishes. If I may borrow a phrase from my daughters, "You guys rock!"

Contents

Introduction   xi

CHAPTER 1: Menopause, Me?—Accepting the Inevitable   1
The Facts: What Is Menopause Anyway?   1
When Will It Happen?   2
What Menopause Means for Your Hormones   5
What's New?   6
Your Body Isn't the Only Thing That's Changing   8
Your Mate May Be Menopausal, Too   9
Why Attitude Matters   12
Talking to Friends and Family   12

CHAPTER 2: Menopause, Then and Now   15
This Isn't Your Mother's Menopause   15
What Your Mother Taught You   15
What Your Mother Taught Medicine   16
Common Wisdom: What's It Worth?   17
Constructing a New Common Wisdom   22
Your Chance for a Brand New Start   24

CHAPTER 3: A Gateway to the Rest of Your Life   25
A Brief History of Menstruation   25
Fast Facts about PMS   27
What Causes Menopause?   29
Taking a Closer Look at Perimenopause   30
Health Concerns   31
Emotional Concerns   33
Social and Family Concerns   34

CHAPTER 4: Perimenopause—Adjusting to the Changes   37
The Journey Through Perimenopause   37
Recognizing the Symptoms   38
Physical Changes   40
Neurological and Cognitive Changes   44
Emotional and Psychological Changes   46
Other Perimenopausal Changes You May Notice   48

CHAPTER 5: Coping with Hot Flashes   51
Hot Flash Facts   51
Techniques for Turning Down the Heat   54
Hormonal Treatments for Hot Flash Relief   55
Nonhormonal Medications   57
Herbs, Botanicals, and Other Alternatives   59
Mind-Body Exercises   61

CHAPTER 6: The New You—Managing Physical Changes   63
Irregular Periods   63
Heavy Bleeding   64
Heart Palpitations   68
Involuntary Urine Release   69
Weight Gain   71
Other Physical Changes Associated with Menopause   73

CHAPTER 7: Managing Cognitive and Neurological Changes 77
My Mind—Where Did it Go?   77
Insomnia and Its Role in Menopause   80
Understanding and Treating Sleep Problems   82
Headaches   86
Dizziness   89
Other Neurological Symptoms   90

**CHAPTER 8: Overcoming Mood Swings, Anxiety, and
Depression   93**
Menopause and Emotions   93
Mood Swings   94
Looking Stress in the Eye   96
Anxiety   99
What Is Depression?   100
Staying "On the Level"   106

**CHAPTER 9: But I'm Still a Woman, Right?—Menopause and
Sexuality   109**
Myths and Fears   109
Checking Your Sexual Attitude   111
The Physical Impact of Changing Hormones   113
Maintaining Your Sexual Health   116
Relationships and Menopause   120
Suggestions for Your Sexual Self—This Could Be Fun!   121

**CHAPTER 10: A Partner on the Path—Choosing a
Health Provider   125**
Do You Have the Provider You Need Now?   125
Personal Qualities of Your Health Care Provider   126
Professional Qualifications   128
Finding the Right Fit   131
Talk with Your Doctor   133
Take an Active Role   136
Listen Up, Speak Up, Be Honest   137

CHAPTER 11: Deciding Whether Hormone Therapy Is
Right for You   139
The Role of Hormones in Your Health   139
The Facts about MHT   146
MHT Options   149
Designer Estrogens   152
Weighing Risks and Benefits   153
Part of a Healthy Menopause Plan   154

CHAPTER 12: Alternatives to MHT   157
Why Some Women Choose MHT Alternatives   157
Nonhormonal Medications   159
Choosing Natural Alternatives Wisely   163
Herbs and Other Supplements   165
Plant Estrogens   169
Therapeutic Programs   172

CHAPTER 13: Health Risks after Forty   175
The Health Risks You Face after Forty   175
Heart Disease   176
Cancer Risks   178
Osteoporosis   185
Urinary Tract Disorders and Yeast Infections   186
Assessing Your Health History   189

CHAPTER 14: Menopause and Heart Disease   191
What Is Heart Disease?   191
The Symptoms of Heart Disease   192
Women, Menopause, and Heart Disease   194
Risk Factors You Can't Change   198
Risks You Can Influence   199
Controlling Your Risks   206

CHAPTER 15: Maintaining Bone Health   207
Close-Up on Osteoporosis   207
What to Watch For   209
Menopause and Osteoporosis   211
Understanding and Controlling Your Risks   213
Eating for Strong Bones   214
Beyond Diet: Measures to Prevent Bone Loss   217

CHAPTER 16: Eating for a Healthy Menopause   223
Your Nutritional Needs after Forty   223
Nutritional Boosts for Women over Forty   225

Get It from Your Plate, Not a Pill 228
Eating for Weight Management 229
Sane, Simple Guidelines for Healthy Eating 234
Your Own Revolution 236

CHAPTER 17: Building Exercise into Your Menopause Plan 237
Why You Need Exercise Now 237
Exercise Can Save Your Life 239
Managing Symptoms of Menopause 241
What Kind of Exercise Do You Need? 244
Choosing an Exercise Program 249
Helpful Workouts 250
Excercise for Life 251

CHAPTER 18: Keeping Your Mind Sharp 253
How Your Brain Changes as You Age 253
Give Your Brain the Nutrition It Needs 255
Exercise Your Body to Keep Your Brain Healthy 255
Exercise Your Brain to Keep It Lively 256
New Activities and Plenty of Rest: Recipe for
a Sharp Mind 258
Methods to Enhance Your Memory 260

CHAPTER 19: Taking Care of All of You 263
Appreciating the Woman in the Mirror 263
Changes in Vision 264
Protecting Your Hearing 268
Keeping Teeth Healthy 269
Caring for Your Skin and Hair 271
Making Time for Rest and Relaxation 276

CHAPTER 20: Can Being Older Mean Being Happier? 279
The Role of a Healthy Body and Mind 279
Stress and Loss 281
Perspective Shifts after Fifty 283
Contributing to Your World 285
Living for the Rest of Your Life 287
Be Creative! 289

Appendix A: Glossary 291
Appendix B: Keeping a Menopause Journal 299
Appendix C: References and Resources 303
Appendix D: Your After-Forty Health Maintenance Plan 309

Index 315

Introduction

Despite its reputation, menopause is more than just some annoying phase that women go through. Like puberty, it is a physical marker that ushers you into a new stage of your life, and (like puberty) it requires time and information to understand all the changes. If you are a woman experiencing the hormone swings and changes that accompany menopause, then the more you know about what's coming, the better you will be able to take charge of your transition.

There is plenty of information about menopause available, and it can be confusing and contradictory. There are books, Web sites, magazine articles, and medical journals all offering bits and pieces of information to enlighten you on this important topic. Sorting through it can be not only frustrating, but confusing and overwhelming. *The Everything®* *Health Guide to Menopause* collects many of those pieces of information in a user-friendly and organized way so that you can explore the topics that interest you and learn about menopause in plain language. Whether you are curious about osteoporosis or hormone therapy, you will find it here. And even some of those questions that are hard to ask your doctor, like "Will I still be able to enjoy sex?" or "Why am I a blubbering idiot some days?" are explained, along with some strategies for dealing with them.

Although the basics of healthy menopause boil down to the basics of all healthy lifestyles—exercise, diet, sleep, and state of mind—this book explores them as they relate to your journey through that last reproductive hurdle. It offers you choices for improving your health and well being, and ideas for making menopause the beginning of an exciting and enriching time. You have a continuing opportunity for improving your life, and menopause is the perfect excuse to take stock and make the changes you've been meaning to make for years.

The baby boomers have had an enormous impact on American life in their every stage of development. As children they required more and better schools; as young adults they redefined sexual expectations and intimacy; as a workforce they have changed the landscape of "work environment"; and it only stands to reason that they will change our collective outlook on getting older. With so many women approaching menopause, there will be more attention to this important stage of life, and there is already more research and information than ever before on women's health over the lifespan. If you are approaching menopause or in the midst of it, you are in a lot of good company.

Using the chapters in this book to educate yourself on the process of menopause will give you ideas about how to talk to your health care provider about what matters to you. Are hot flashes making you crazy? Are you embarrassed to tell your doctor that you wet your pants when you laugh? These are legitimate concerns that can be addressed and treated, and this book can give you the information you need to discuss these and other common menopausal complaints with your health care provider.

Above all, you need support and knowledge. You need information that teaches you about menopause and that helps you make the right choices for you. Keeping your perspective during a time of hormone shifts and life changes is no small matter. And keeping your health as you move through menopause and beyond will make the transition not a dreaded ordeal, but rather the open door to the rest of your life.

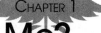

CHAPTER 1

Menopause, Me?— Accepting the Inevitable

MENOPAUSE IS A TOPIC some women would rather ignore than explore. Many younger women see it as "irrelevant," but as they approach the age of menopause they look around for reassurance that it is not only survivable, but something to look forward to. The bad press may leave you worried or confused, but before you deny it, despair at it or try to dodge it, let's take a look at what menopause really is.

The Facts: What Is Menopause Anyway?

The simple answer is this: Menopause is when your period finally stops. But because your periods may become less regular and occur at greater intervals as you approach menopause, you don't know you've gone through menopause until twelve months have passed since your last period.

Count the Months

According to the Council of Affiliated Menopause Societies (CAMS), menopause is "The permanent end of menstruation. Menopause is not a disease but a natural event in a woman's life that results from a decrease in the ovarian production of sex hormones—estrogen, progesterone, and testosterone. Menopause is confirmed when a woman has not had a menstrual period for twelve consecutive months." By the time you know you've experienced natural menopause, you're already saying, "So *that* was menopause?"

How Menopause Affects You

Menopause doesn't make a grand entrance—no fanfare, no fireworks. Menopause becomes a reality for most women through a series of physical, mental, and emotional changes—some subtle, some more dramatic—that tend to emerge, evolve, intensify, and fade over a period of weeks, months, and years. What most women refer to as "menopause," with symptoms such as hot flashes, memory problems, and mood swings, is actually the period leading up to menopause, called perimenopause. The changes are unique to each individual, so women don't have a single "menopause profile" to compare themselves to. Menopause can have many faces, and there's no one best way to prepare for or experience it. And it's not as bad as you may think!

 Alert

> To avoid unnecessary worry and discomfort about menopause, don't deny the obvious. Learn all you can about what's happening to your body, and then take the necessary next steps to begin making your passage through menopause as painless and productive as you possibly can. You've made a great start by picking up this book!

When Will It Happen?

Predicting when you will go through your menopause is definitely not an exact science. According to the North American Menopause Society (NAMS), the average age of natural menopause in the Western world is fifty-one. This of course is only an average, and women may experience menopause when they are as young as thirty, or well into their sixties. The good news about menopause is that the end of childbearing can mean the beginning of other sorts of productivity. With more leisure time, older, independent children, and a perspective broadened by experience, women can begin to engage in satisfying activities that they have either abandoned with the onset of responsibilities, or never been able to explore. Since most American women born after 1950 can expect to live until their mid-eighties, the majority of menopausal women in the United States today have one-half to one-third of their lives to live after they've gone through menopause. Many factors determine your age at menopause, including which type of menopause you experience.

Natural Menopause

As its name implies, natural menopause refers to the natural process of ceasing to menstruate. It occurs as your ovaries stop producing hormones, and usually occurs between the ages of forty-eight and fifty-five, with the average at about fifty-one and a half years.

Induced Menopause

Induced menopause occurs when a woman has her ovaries surgically removed (with or without a total hysterectomy) or when ovaries stop functioning as a result of chemotherapy, radiation, drug therapy, or other medical treatments. Because induced menopause is the result of unexpected physical conditions or deliberate health decisions such as surgery or chemotherapy, it can happen at any age.

Whenever induced menopause is a possible side effect of medical care, it should be discussed with your medical provider so that you can prepare yourself for the sudden change in hormone levels. Because the onset of induced menopause is so abrupt, there is no gradual adjustment period to prepare for postmenopausal changes. Women who have had both ovaries surgically removed, for example, may experience dramatic, abrupt menopausal symptoms.

Essential

Having a hysterectomy doesn't mean you'll go through menopause. If your uterus is removed but your ovaries remain, your body will continue to produce hormones. In this case, you don't experience menopause as a result of your surgery, even though you won't have monthly menstrual bleeding. On the other hand, women who have a surgical menopause (ovaries removed) have a more sudden hormone change and don't have the same time to adjust to the changes. Their symptoms may be more dramatic!

Hysterectomy

Surgical removal of the uterus alone will not cause menopause as long as the ovaries remain in place and are not damaged by the surgery. What does disappear, however, is the visible signal that you are going through menopause—changes in your monthly cycle. While you stop bleeding each month—often a welcome effect of surgery—you may not realize that your perimenopause is underway.

Chemotherapy

Chemotherapy, the use of drugs to treat cancer, may not result in immediate menopause, but it can damage the ovaries. Depending upon the types of drugs your treatment involves, your ovaries might recover and function normally some time after treatment ends. In some cases, chemotherapy damages ovaries so severely that they cannot produce adequate amounts of hormones. In those cases, menopause may occur months or even years after the therapy has ended. Doctors can't always predict whether damaged ovaries will recover.

Radiation

Pelvic radiation therapy can cause permanent ovarian failure (and therefore, premature menopause) when the ovaries are the target of high doses of radiation, for example, as treatment for cervical cancer. Since radiation therapy is a tightly targeted therapy, it often has no effect on ovarian function. If ovaries receive only low doses of radiation, they're likely to fully recover their functions.

Other Factors Influencing the Timing of Menopause

There are some factors that may influence the timing of your menopause. Often women will go through menopause at the same age as their mothers or sisters do, suggesting a genetic link to the timing. If you are overweight or have had more than one pregnancy, you may experience menopause a bit later than you would have otherwise. On the other hand, if you have never had a baby, if you have cardiac disease, or if you were treated for certain types of childhood cancer, you may have your menopause earlier. And if you are a smoker, you may experience menopause as much as two years earlier than if you hadn't smoked at all.

What Menopause Means for Your Hormones

Your body produces dozens of hormones, but three of them play a major role in your reproductive cycle. Those three are estrogen, progesterone, and small quantities of androgens (testosterone, for example).

Each hormone has a job to do. The three types of hormones that affect your cycle have distinctive roles to play:

- Estrogen is a growth hormone that stimulates the development of adult sex organs during puberty; helps retain calcium in bones; regulates the balance of "good" and "bad" cholesterol in the bloodstream; and aids other body functions, such as blood sugar level, memory functions, and emotional balance.
- Progesterone balances the effects of estrogen. It aids the maturation of body tissues and limits their growth; stimulates the uterus, breasts, and fallopian tubes to secrete nutrients necessary for the body to prepare for growing an embryo and bearing a child; and raises both body temperature and blood sugar levels.
- Androgens are male hormones produced in small quantities by the ovaries and adrenal glands—with the greatest quantities occurring at the midpoint of a woman's cycle—that contribute to a healthy libido by fostering a desire for sex.

Essential

As the frequency of your ovulation decreases, the follicle-stimulating hormone (FSH) levels in your bloodstream increase. In fact, your doctor can test the level of FSH in your blood to determine if it is elevated, which may indicate that you are nearing menopause and may be helpful in determining fertility. There are also home test kits to measure this hormone in your urine.

Lower Hormones Equal Big Changes

If each hormone plays such an important role in your reproductive life, what happens when the levels begin to drop? That is a complicated question, and the short answer is: menopause. But as a woman goes through the menopausal years, the changes in these hormone levels cause many changes in her body and in her life. This book is all about such changes and how to deal with them. For each woman it will be a different story, and her approach will be different depending on her specific response to these changes.

What's New?

Now that Baby Boomers are entering into menopause and postmeno-pause it is being studied as never before. There are 38 million "boomer" women between the ages of forty and fifty-eight. This generation of women who were never going to "trust anyone over thirty" are having understandable struggles with accepting the aging process. The good news is that resources are now being devoted to studying the health risks of the menopausal years.

The Women's Health Initiative (WHI) Study

In 1992, the landmark Women's Health Initiative (WHI) study was launched by the National Heart, Lung, and Blood Institute (NHLBI) of the National Institutes of Health (NIH). This study is the largest long-term study of menopausal women's health ever done in the United States and focuses on the major causes of death and disability in postmenopausal women. It includes over 161,000 women from diverse racial and ethnic backgrounds from around the country, and provides scientific and practical information on the causes and risks of chronic disease so that women and their care providers can make informed choices.

Hormone Therapies

For decades, it was accepted medical practice to offer women some sort of hormone replacement therapy to ease the transition into post-menopause and to lower the risks associated with the transition, such as cancer, heart disease, and osteoporosis. One of the most dramatic results from the WHI study was the discovery that not only is estrogen replacement not always protective, it may even *increase* the risk of disease in female patients. These remarkable findings caused confusion in the medical community about the wisdom of menopausal hormone therapies, and follow-up studies are still sorting out the risks and details.

Exercise

Exercise has long been recommended for general health improvement, and menopause only underlines the value of it for women. New research shows just how important exercise can be for improving not only general health, but also quality of life and reduction of many menopausal symptoms. It affects mood, flexibility, bone density, joint comfort, heart health, and cancer risk. And you don't have to be a marathon runner or triathelete to benefit from adopting exercise into your routine. Many types of activity—from strength training to simple walking—can make noticeable improvements in your menopausal health. Knowing the facts can help you make good choices about the type of exercise that will work for you.

Sexuality

It's not too surprising that the generation that authored "The Sexual Revolution" seems determined to continue the pleasures of a healthy sex life. With the development of drugs for erectile dysfunction and increased focus on women's sexual response, sexual activity is seen as a normal part of life well into later years. Menopause can have a marked impact on your approach to this aspect of your life as mood changes, vaginal dryness, and decreased libido begin to rear their heads. Managing these and other symptoms is acceptable now that women are voicing their dissatisfaction with their sex lives around menopause. Research in the areas of sexuality offers hope and choices for making this a free and satisfying time of life for you and your partner. Chapter 9 explores sexuality during and after menopause and provides information and resources to keep your sexual self thriving.

Chronic Disease

As women move through the menopause and on to the rest of life, they are at increasing risk for chronic diseases like diabetes, heart disease, cancer, and arthritis. With the right attitude and information, you can minimize these risks and make simple lifestyle changes that can make an enormous difference in your quality of life and even your lifespan! As research focuses on the differences between women's health and men's health, it is clear that many health conditions can be minimized or prevented if you learn about them early.

Your Body Isn't the Only Thing That's Changing

Most perimenopausal and early postmenopausal women today are Baby Boomers, and some of them are Generation Xers (born between 1961 and 1981). These graying generations are among the largest and most influential of the current U.S. population, and they're taking America with them through the menopause experience. If you're in perimenopause or have experienced menopause, you're certainly not alone.

Many women today enter their most productive years after the age of forty. Careers are established, children more independent, and a stronger sense of self emerges. Women begin to care less about what others think; inner strength and self-awareness blossom. Although youth and beauty are often considered inseparable, cultural ideas about beauty are changing to include older women. Women are seeing themselves as attractive into their later years, and this attractiveness contributes to the growing self-confidence that often accompanies this period.

But most women of forty are also approaching a decade of dramatic personal, physical, and psychosocial change, a new stage of life that may be occurring at a time when they may be uninterested in—and maybe even resistant to—preparing for it. As personal as each woman's perimenopause may be, no woman is alone as she enters this phase of her life.

 Fact

According the U.S. Census data, there are about 37.5 million women at or near menopause (age forty to fifty-nine). Every year, the population gets proportionately "grayer"—so don't worry, you have lots of company!

Your Kids Are Maturing

Other women your age aren't your only companions in incredible change during these years. If you have children in your mid- to late twenties or early thirties, by the time you begin experiencing the first signs of perimenopause, it's quite likely that your children may be going through puberty and adolescence.

You went through puberty, so you know what your kids are going through when they reach adolescence. Their bodies and minds are in turmoil. As kids pass through relatively rapid physical changes (some they see as good, others horrify them), they also begin that important first round of "Who am I?" introspection and exploration. They may feel confused, angry, loving, hateful, homely, childlike, adultlike, happy, depressed, bored, excited, and lonely—and that's all just in the first fifteen minutes after they wake up in the morning. If you think the dynamic of an adolescent's raging hormones can wreak havoc on a household, what about combining that loaded pistol with the fluctuating hormonal shifts of a perimenopausal mother?

When you and your child are both trying to figure out who you are and what you want from life, even as you're trying to cope with changing physical and mental patterns in your life, the atmosphere is ripe for conflict.

Of course, you also have a rare opportunity to connect with your child on a whole new level that women who aren't experiencing perimenopause are unlikely to enjoy. But doing this requires a great deal of effort, patience, and creativity on your part. You may or may not be able to turn this dual passage into a positive phase in your family's development, but it's certainly worth a try. You might want to take this opportunity to realize that you and your child are both going through big changes simultaneously and that this is an opportunity to connect with your children on that level.

Your Mate May Be Menopausal, Too

You don't have to be in a same-sex relationship to experience couple's menopause. Though the phenomenon of male menopause was first the subject of research in the 1940s, even twenty years ago you would have had to search for scientific references to male menopause. Today, the medical and psychological communities treat the subject with much more respect.

 Alert

> Don't feel put off if other women in your family didn't (or don't) share your signs and symptoms. Every woman is unique in her perimenopausal experience—even within her own family.

Men Have Their Own Change

You've probably heard the worn-out jokes about men going through a midlife crisis—a syndrome that somehow manifests itself in the form of a hairpiece, a twenty-something trophy wife, or a shiny red sports car. Well, many men do experience a psychosocial passage known as a midlife crisis, triggered by flagging sexuality, career plateaus, and the realization that "having it all" isn't all it was cracked up to be. But that midlife event, as important as it may be, isn't the same as male menopause.

Male menopause, known as andropause in the medical community, reportedly affects nearly 40 percent of men between the ages of forty and sixty. All men begin producing less testosterone after the age of forty. As testosterone levels decrease, men may find that they experience fewer erections, that the erections are more difficult to sustain, and that they experience longer intervals between erections. Male menopause can result in a wide range of symptoms in men including lethargy, depression, mood swings, insomnia, hot flashes, irritability, and decreased sexual desire.

Diminishing testosterone in the bloodstream isn't the only culprit behind male menopause. Other factors include obesity, excess alcohol consumption, hypertension and the medications used to treat it, lack of exercise, and other "middle-age plagues" that damage health. While medications have been developed to treat erectile dysfunction, testosterone therapy is one of the few non-behavioral medical treatments available for combating male menopause.

Fact

Sexual dysfunction isn't the only marker of male menopause. Studies show that nearly 51 percent of men ages forty to seventy experience some level of impotence in varying degrees of severity and persistence—and that's many more than the number who exhibit symptoms of male menopause.

Two Women Does Not Equal an Easy Time

If you are in a same-sex relationship, the chances are very good that at some point you and your mate may both be experiencing symptoms of approaching menopause. Although it may seem that sharing a household with another menopausal woman could lead to increased conflict, you also have a life-partner who may be better able to understand your experience. Both of you will need to remember, however, that every woman's menopause experience is unique, so neither of you can expect the other to have the same symptoms or reactions to those symptoms.

So what does this have to do with your passage through perimenopause and menopause?

If you and your mate are both experiencing the mood swings, irritability, and other negative effects of menopause at the same time, both of you may have a rougher time dealing with the experience. Your partner may or may not understand or accept her own struggle with midlife passage, and that could put extra demands on your patience and understanding—at a time when you won't feel particularly well endowed with either. The message here is that your partner may not have the reserves of patience and support necessary to help you through all of the rough patches of menopause, and at times you may have to draw on your deepest supply of those qualities to avoid throwing gasoline on the smoldering fires of family discord.

Why Attitude Matters

At no previous time in history has society known more about both the biology and psychology of menopause and aging. There have never been as many therapeutic options for taming the symptoms of menopause. People now have an unprecedented understanding of diet and nutrition and the roles they play in healthy aging.

Pay Attention to Your Notions

As you approach menopause, you may not have evaluated your attitude toward the transition you are making. The way you think about menopause, aging, change, and your own self-worth is vital at this time of physical and emotional transition. There is a growing body of research showing that "expectation physiology" has enormous impact on outcome. What you think is what you get! While it may be easy to believe the worst about menopause, it's also possible to see menopause for what it is—and what it can be.

Rearrange Your Thinking

Now is your chance to evaluate some of the "truths" you've learned about menopause and aging over the years, and how those ideas can affect your attitude toward your own experience. You can also take a closer look at some of the myths and fears that surround menopause even in today's enlightened social climate and learn some simple techniques for tracking unhealthy beliefs to their source and cleaning them out of your mental closet.

Talking to Friends and Family

Old schools of thought tell you that, like a fairy tale monster that feeds on fear, menopause exists only in the imagination and is best defeated by denying its existence. According to this philosophy, you won't have any problems with perimenopause if you simply ignore it. Nice try, but perimenopause doesn't really work that way.

Perimenopause and menopause are real medical and psychological events, with some actual indicators and symptoms. Perimenopause is unique to each woman, so no one can know what you're feeling and experiencing during this time. You may experience no symptoms of perimenopause, or you may have hot flashes or mood swings that you are certain everyone around you must notice. Bottling up your feelings and trying to hide your perimenopausal symptoms from your family or your close friends may seem like the best thing for them, but in fact it's unlikely to help anyone—particularly you—understand and deal with the realities of this time in your life.

One of the most important things you can do to make your perimenopausal experience sane and healthy (for you and your family) is to communicate openly with them about your physical and emotional condition. Talk about your symptoms and how they affect your mood, concentration, ability to sleep, level of anxiety, or whatever applies to your experience. Answer their questions and ask for their understanding. If perimenopause is making you irritable and impatient, try to establish some mutual rules for resolving family issues and avoiding unnecessary conflicts. Ask those you care about to help you find a way for everyone to move through the experience and emerge in one piece.

When It's a Family Affair

If you're sharing a life-changing moment with your child, you're going to have to be patient, strong, and attentive. Your spouse or partner may have to step in and take a more active role in parenting, to relieve you of some of the stress and responsibility during certain phases of your perimenopausal changes. You may find that you need a mediator to work through some family difficulties—a relative, counselor, teacher, or family friend.

You and your mate may have to spend more time listening to each other and learning new patterns of behavior. Things are evolving in your life and, therefore, in your relationship. Take this opportunity to revisit the way you think about your lover, life-mate, partner, and friend and to begin interacting with that person on a deeper, more meaningful level.

You can rest assured that your mother and older female relatives have shared at least some portion of your experience in perimenopause. This experience may offer an opportunity to relate to your family in entirely new ways—and, with any luck, at least some of those ways will be positive!

Give Everyone a Break

Most importantly, try not to waste time judging yourself or your loved ones on the success rate of your communications and relationships during this time. If perimenopause teaches anything, it is that you continue to be a work in progress. Every day will offer new challenges and perhaps some new insights and opportunities to learn something about yourself, your family, your coworkers, and the ways you interact with all of them. If you cut yourself a little slack—accept the fact that once in a while you won't feel and act exactly as you may wish you could—you're more likely to give those around you a little more breathing room, too. Everybody's learning as they go; but when you enter perimenopause, your body signals to you that your life lessons are about to become much more interesting.

CHAPTER 2

Menopause, Then and Now

A WOMAN ENTERING MENOPAUSE TODAY has much more information than in generations past. She has Internet access, new research, media coverage, and health care providers to help her understand her choices. But along with this updated information, she may have some outdated ideas about what menopause means. This chapter will explore the difference between the past meaning of menopause and how it has changed in recent years. It will help you understand some of the myths and common misunderstandings about menopause, and how you can develop your own understanding to this life stage.

This Isn't Your Mother's Menopause

Women's attitudes about menopause, and the ability to communicate about it, are often shaped by their generation. When your mother was born, little was said about menopause, and few women would have felt comfortable talking about "the change" even within a group of friends. Today, it's not unusual for menopause to be the subject of happy hour chatter. So, while the conversation about menopause has changed, how about the way we think about menopause? Have ideas and beliefs about menopause gone through a true evolution?

What Your Mother Taught You

If you ask many women in their fifties today what their mothers told them about menopause, they're likely to respond, "She never mentioned it to me." Although it appeared that the 1970s and 80s would break down the barriers that deemed menopause an unacceptable topic, there was still very little good information available about menopause until recently. Your mother couldn't teach you what she didn't know herself.

Wanted: Good Research

Much of the lack of new information about menopause during this time was the result of a shortage of good research prior to the last quarter of the twentieth century. And the research that was being conducted wasn't available to the general public; these were pre-Internet years, remember, and newspapers and television shows weren't likely to report new findings in the field of menopause. So, many women in the 1970s didn't have access to updated, comprehensive medical information about symptoms, their cause, and how they might be alleviated.

Unspoken Attitudes Can Still Be Absorbed

Though your mother may have never discussed menopause with you, that doesn't mean you didn't "inherit" certain beliefs about menopause. Your mother's beliefs about menopause—and the general attitude of the women in her generation—were probably transferred to you, whether or not those beliefs were spoken. How your mother handled menopause has likely colored your attitude—and will, therefore, help shape your experience.

What Your Mother Taught Medicine

Since the late 1970s, the medical profession has studied menopausal women more than in any time in history, and what it has learned from those women—a group that includes the mothers of baby boomers—has changed the way our culture views menopause.

Not Just "In Your Head"

Symptoms such as hot flashes, insomnia, and irritability were once viewed as all-in-the-head responses to the panic of aging. Today, many scientists trace these symptoms to specific changes in hormone levels. In the 1980s, most women viewed hormone replacement therapy (HRT) as the only option for relieving menopausal symptoms. Today, hormone therapy is just one treatment choice. The world is a different place for today's menopausal women thanks, in part, to data gathered for and by their mothers' generation.

More Information and Choices

Today there is a wide variety of health care resources, treatment options, support groups, information sources, and discussion forums to turn to for information, advice, and ideas about having a healthy menopause. Menopausal women don't have to "shut up and get through it" or deny that they're experiencing natural emotional and physical reactions to this important passage. Today's fifty-year-olds have one-third of their lives ahead of them. They will live longer than any generation of women that preceded them, and they won't experience this "third age" as their mothers experienced it. To live the years ahead productively and happily, women in this group must come face to face with their body, their health, and their attitudes toward menopause.

Common Wisdom: What's It Worth?

Sex education has changed a lot over the years. You may recall the plastic model of the female reproductive organs that graced the teacher's desk. At some point in the course, the teacher would send the model around the room, so everyone could get a closer look. The girls would pass the model around, eyeing it casually and handing it to the next student—nothing to see here, folks! The sexual revolution was just unfolding, and young girls were learning to regard their bodies and sexuality in whole new ways.

In a time of growing sexual freedom, baby boomers learned to be cool and nonchalant about sexuality—and they certainly weren't caught up in issues their mothers and grandmothers thought of as "female problems." They laughed at old euphemisms for menstruation, such as "falling off the roof" or "getting the curse." In an age of feminism, these women learned to toss aside old concepts of feminine weakness and fragility and recognize themselves as strong, capable, freethinking, sexual creatures.

But now, as they approach menopause, many women in this postfeminist age are considering their femaleness from another perspective. At some point, every woman begins to contemplate certain facts about this time of transition, and to acknowledge some of the following basic truths:

- Some physical aspects of the aging process are unique to women.
- The body and mind of a fifty-year-old woman is different from that of a twenty-five-year-old woman.
- Menopause marks a physical change in a woman's body, and every woman's reaction to that physical change will be different.

Beyond these simple, basic truths, however, most people hold a number of ideas and attitudes toward menopause and aging—some true and some false. So how do you think about menopause? Do you dread it? Are you looking forward to the freedom of moving beyond menstruation and into a life free of unwanted pregnancy? Or do you equate fertility with femininity, and worry that menopause will leave you dried up and dreary? Are you hopeful that with the right diet, treatment plan, and nutritional supplements you can get back the body you had at twenty-five? Or at least keep the one you have at forty-five? Do you know the woman you are, and can you accept the woman you are becoming?

Your attitude toward menopause and the aging process will determine the answers to many of these questions. And the first step in understanding how you feel about menopause is to examine the source of those feelings and ideas. The common wisdom of menopause—the information and misinformation that fuels society's beliefs—plays an important role in determining what people believe. So, take a moment to review some of the beliefs that make up the common wisdom of menopause, so you can understand the truths—and untruths—they hold.

Myth #1: Menopausal Women Lose Interest in Sex

The lack-of-libido mythology about women in menopause is part of the common wisdom shared by both men and women—and it's simply not true. Masters and Johnson conducted a study that demonstrated no link between estrogen levels and libido. A number of studies have shown that only a small percentage of postmenopausal women report a lack of interest in sex, and over half of all women studied report no decrease in sexual interest at all after menopause. In fact, the American

Association of Retired Persons (AARP) *Modern Maturity* Sexual Survey, conducted in 1999 and repeated in 2004, showed over half of men and women age forty-five and older say they're satisfied with their sex lives, and many say they enjoy sex "now more than ever." In the 2004 survey, women reported that when their male partners used medication for erectile dysfunction, the men's increased satisfaction enhanced the women's satisfaction as well.

So where did this myth come from? The truth is that women suffering from severe estrogen depletion can experience some discomfort during sex due to drier, thinner, less flexible vaginal walls and occasional itching and burning near the vaginal opening. A woman experiencing hot flashes, disturbed sleep patterns, headaches, and other occasional symptoms of menopause is unlikely to feel as sexually eager as she would otherwise. However, none of these conditions is permanent or untreatable, and many of them aren't inevitable, either. So if you believe that menopause equals the end of sex as you know it, you're wrong.

 ## Fact

Authors Leah Kliger and Deborah Nedelman are doing their share to construct a new "common wisdom" in their book, *Still Sexy After All These Years?: The 9 Unspoken Truths About Women's Desire Beyond 50.* Their research supports the notion that women not only remain sexually vital after fifty but sometimes feel more sexually fulfilled than at any other time in their lives.

Myth #2: Menopausal Women Gain Weight, Have Hot Flashes, and Lose Control of Their Emotions

Lots of people think that the typical woman in menopause is fat, flushed, and out of control. While hot flashes, weight gain, and mood swings are all symptoms reported by some women in menopause, they aren't inevitable side effects of the passage. In fact, many women—as many as 10 to 20 percent of women studied—exhibit no symptoms of menopause at all. And while studies show that as many as half of all women in perimenopause experience some weight gain, other women actually lose weight during perimenopause; and many of those who gain weight before menopause lose it afterward (see Chapters 6, 16, and 17 for information about weight management in menopause).

Perhaps as many as 85 percent of menopausal women report hot flashes, but most women find them to be intermittent and, on average, they diminish completely within five years after menopause (see Chapter 5).

Irritability and depression are also symptoms reported by some— but not all—women during perimenopause, but no one should expect depression to be a long-term, ongoing fact of life. In fact, depression is reported at much higher rates among women in their twenties and thirties, and some studies have shown that depression actually decreases in postmenopausal women. And even if you do experience mood swings, they don't have to become part of your identity during menopause (see Chapter 8).

In short, you may or may not have hot flashes, moodiness, and weight gain during menopause—many women don't. But if you do experience these symptoms they are likely to be temporary and can usually be treated.

Myth #3: Hormone Replacement Therapy Is Too Dangerous

Millions of women in menopause use some form of menopausal hormone therapy (MHT), formerly called hormone replacement therapy (HRT). It's true that MHT can have dangerous consequences for women with a history of breast cancer, blood clots, untreated endometrial cancer, and certain other family health concerns. A physician is likely to discourage the use of MHT for women with a history of cancer, and it is definitely not indicated for women with untreated endometrial cancer, but in the end, a careful examination of risks versus the benefits of treating severe menopausal symptoms is the only way to determine a safe, comfortable course of action. Most doctors agree that MHT is one of the most effective methods available today for minimizing both the uncomfortable symptoms (such as hot flashes and vaginal dryness) and health-threatening side effects (including elevated cholesterol levels and bone loss) of menopause. Still, many women continue to view MHT as a treatment option pushed by doctors as a means of making money for both the medical profession and the pharmaceutical industry.

In 2002 the Women's Health Initiative (WHI) study came out with results that seem to show that not only is hormone therapy not protective against some chronic conditions, it may even *increase* the risks for these conditions. Given these results, it halted portions of the study. This brought fear and confusion to patients and clinicians alike. Many women stopped taking their hormones immediately, and physicians began to question what had been common practice.

Further study has shown that while subgroups of patients may be at risk for aggravation of their chronic conditions, many women benefit from some sort of menopause hormone treatment, especially for the common symptoms of hot flashes and vaginal dryness. And these therapies have proven protective in the case of osteoporosis and some types of colon cancer. Each woman has a unique set of risks and symptoms, and the best plan is to discuss your own situation thoroughly with your health provider.

Essential

Many, many studies on the benefits and potential health implications of MHT are underway, and new reports appear regularly. To keep up with some of the latest news about MHT, you can search under "Menopause" on the National Library of Medicine's Web site at *www.nlm.nih.gov/medlineplus/menopause.html*.

You may or may not be a good candidate for MHT, and you certainly can use other methods for treating symptoms. If you do decide to use MHT, you may take it for only a short time. To know and understand your options, read as much as you can on the topic and talk with your doctor and other health care professionals. But keep an open mind, listen to the facts, and learn all you can about MHT (see Chapter 11 for more information). Then make your decision based on fact—not fear.

Myth #4: MHT Is the Only Viable Option for Dealing with the Symptoms of Menopause

MHT isn't the only option for treating menopause symptoms or delaying the aging effects of slowing estrogen production. Depending upon the symptoms you experience, simple lifestyle changes may address your most annoying reminders of perimenopause. Many women in your mother's generation faced a hormone-or-nothing choice. Our understanding of menopause has changed dramatically over the past thirty years.

 Question

What exactly are alternative treatments for symptoms of menopause? Alternative treatments are any treatment other than the traditional treatment of hormone therapy. Alternative treatments include anything from vitamins and herbs, to nutritional supplements of soy and phytoestrogens, to cognitive therapy, acupuncture, and biofeedback.

As women have learned more about the causes and life cycles of certain menopausal symptoms, they feel more comfortable tackling some of them with simple lifestyle changes. You can sleep in a cool bedroom and wear layers of clothing to combat hot flashes, for example. Relaxation therapies can help reduce the occurrence of insomnia, as can changes in eating and drinking habits. If you suffer from anxiety and depression, you might benefit from psychological counseling or biofeedback therapy. A number of herbal remedies, prescription and over-the-counter medications, and dietary supplements are available to help fight off bone loss, high cholesterol, sleeplessness, and other menopause-related health concerns. Women who cannot or prefer not to use estrogen can choose from a number of sound, viable non-MHT treatment options for combating the symptoms of menopause.

Constructing a New Common Wisdom

The previous sections discuss only a few of the commonly held misconceptions about the experience of perimenopause and menopause. While these examples help illustrate how wrong these generalities can be, many other inaccuracies dominate the popular culture about menopause and what it means to go through it. Common wisdom exists because it's easier to accept a set of broad generalizations than it is to dig out the facts. But when it comes to the subject of menopause, generalities that apply in the majority of cases are just not reliable predictors of your experience.

Compare Stories, Find Support

One way to weather the transition through menopause is to find support among women who have gone, or are going, through it. By telling your stories and helping each other understand the process, you can gain a perspective on it and see where you might need to seek treatment and what you might want to ride out. At the very least, you can develop a sense of humor about this phase of your life and take comfort in the fact that you are not alone.

L. Essential

Social groups can teach you a lot about what you are experiencing, and can provide important emotional connection as you navigate the waters of menopause. Get together with your friends during this phase. Start a once-a-month dinner group where you each bring one menopause fact to discuss. Or be the person at work to organize a weekly "flash walk" where women can get outdoors and talk with each other about how menopause is affecting each of you.

Chart Your Own Course

Every woman's experience in menopause will differ. And yours is really the only experience that matters to you. If you keep an open mind and pay attention to your own body, you'll find your own set of common wisdom truths about this transition and what it means for you. If you monitor and respond to your own reactions and discuss your concerns openly and thoroughly with your health care provider, you'll be able to make the best lifestyle and health care decisions for you.

Your Chance for a Brand New Start

If women in the past thought of menopause as the beginning of the end, more and more women today are seizing upon this time of transition as an opportunity to make important changes in their lifestyles and behavior. As mentioned earlier, many women devote their premenopausal adult years to focusing outward, on the demands of family, finances, and careers. As a woman approaches menopause, however, her life may offer her many new opportunities for personal freedom and growth. Many postmenopausal women find that their family and home lives actually improve at this time and that they have a greater sense of personal fulfillment.

From "Reproductive" to "Productive"

With less time spent caring for young children, or developing first-time relationships with husbands or partners, or gaining a foothold in the workplace, postmenopausal women can devote more time to their personal interests. Women find new energy and interest in returning to pursuits they abandoned in their twenties and thirties, including creative outlets such as painting, writing, and photography. Many women at the age of menopause find themselves able to devote time and energy to travel, finishing an abandoned academic degree, or starting a new business.

Menopause is a time when many women make important lifestyle changes. During most of your life, you may not have worried much about issues such as nutrition and exercise or the health-threatening impact of smoking, living with stress, or inadequate sleep. But as you approach the age of menopause, you may find that you're ready to make changes in your habits in order to ensure a happier, healthier future. In fact, though the stereotype of age may be that it's a time of reminiscence and living in the past, many women find themselves contemplating the future more than ever as they approach menopause. Though you may be nearing the end of your reproductive years, your productivity may achieve levels you've never known.

CHAPTER 3

A Gateway to the Rest of Your Life

MENOPAUSE IS THE GATE through which you pass to the next third of your life. It has been preceded by other phases that have set the stage for your next decades. This chapter will look at the phases you have already passed through, and will take a closer look at the perimenopause as you prepare to find your way through yet another life-altering stage.

A Brief History of Menstruation

Women in their teens, twenties, and early thirties usually experience regular monthly menstrual cycles. Some people label this time frame "the reproductive years," but it's important to remember that as long as you ovulate and have periods, you are fertile and you can conceive. For the purposes of this book, therefore, just think of that life stage as that of early adulthood, which lasts, for the average woman, into her forties.

By the time most women reach their late teens, they ovulate regularly, and their bodies establish their "normal" reproductive cycle. Although the length and regularity of the monthly cycle varies from woman to woman, you can think of the typical reproductive cycle as occurring in two main phases:

- **Buildup**—(follicular phase), the time when the ovaries begin developing a group of follicles, each containing an egg, starting on the first day of menstrual bleeding and continuing until midway through the cycle when one egg has become fully developed and ovulation occurs. This is also the time that the uterine lining begins to thicken again after it is shed with menstruation.
- **Premenstrual**—(secretory phase), the time following ovulation when the uterine lining matures and prepares for the implantation of a potential fertilized egg.

Every month, through a complex series of hormonal changes, you get ready to be pregnant. Then, if you aren't, you shed the lining of your uterus and start all over again. You know this as your menstrual cycle and, love it or hate it, it has marked the passage of time since the day you started your first period.

Here are some helpful terms for discussing your periods:

- **Menstruation, menses, and menorrhea:** Terms for the monthly bleeding that you call your period
- **Menarche:** The beginning of menstruation marked by your first menstrual period
- **Amenorrhea:** Absence of periods
- **Dysmenorrhea:** Painful periods

Menarche: The Beginning

In the United States, the average age of a girl's first period is twelve years old, but you may have started anywhere from age eight to age sixteen, and it would still be considered normal. The timing of your first period is determined by a number of things, including whether you were well nourished, the age of your mother's first period, whether you had enough body fat to start the necessary hormone production, and whether you were ill or had certain birth defects. You probably remember the day of your first period and can recall how people around you reacted to the event. This was the beginning of your outlook on menstruation, and even formed some of your ideas about being a woman.

Your Periods

If you are approaching menopause age, you have been having periods for almost thirty years! By now you have formed some pretty strong ideas about what those periods mean to you. Do you call it "The Curse?" Or do you see it as the hallmark of being a woman? What does fertility mean to you? Does it mean monthly pain, or the chance to have your wonderful children? Or both?

You probably have had a cycle somewhere between twenty-one and thirty-five days long, and have bled from four to seven days each time.

These fertile years have been a defining part of you for your entire adult life. Fertility can be the cause of pain or joy, sometimes in the same day. As menopause appears on the horizon, you will have to adjust your way of thinking about yourself.

Beyond what your periods mean to you as a woman, you have also learned how they affect your everyday life. Maybe your personality changes during different parts of the month, maybe you are more interested in sex mid-cycle and not at all immediately before your period, or maybe you are even-tempered and easy going all month long. All of these are normal, and by now you can pretty well predict what is normal for you. With the upcoming changes of menopause this may all be turned on its head. You may become unpredictable to yourself, having to learn about your new body and change your expectations of yourself. Something like adolescence, but without the growth spurt.

Ⅼ. Essential

According to some studies, your menstrual cycles may shorten sometime around age forty, then lengthen slightly as you approach menopause. So, while your period may occur every twenty-six days when you're forty years old, as you reach forty-five, thirty-five-day cycles may become normal for you.

Fast Facts about PMS

Even when you've established your own individual cycle and are in the height of your reproductive years—from your late twenties through mid-thirties—your monthly cycle may not be a smooth ride. Most women experience some symptoms around their menstrual periods including cramps, swollen and tender breasts, mood shifts, and headaches. These symptoms can also happen—along with others—in premenstrual syndrome (PMS). Some research indicates that PMS can include as many as 150 separate systems, but all symptoms of PMS fall into two major categories:

- Physical symptoms of PMS include bloating, water retention, pelvic pressure or cramping, clumsiness, and headaches or migraines.
- Emotional symptoms can consist of irritability, anxiety, mood swings, difficulty concentrating, and food cravings.

The Many Degrees of PMS

Some women never have PMS, while others—some studies estimate as many as 75 percent of all women—may have episodes of it throughout their adult lives. These women often find that PMS is more frequent and severe during their thirties. On the other hand, some women who have never experienced PMS or have had only occasional minor symptoms, report severe PMS phases as they enter perimenopause.

 Alert

Although PMS symptoms can occur anywhere from midway through your cycle to the day you begin your period, no one symptom should ever last more than two weeks (by definition, if symptoms occur after the start of your period, it may not be PMS). If you have any symptom longer than fourteen days, or symptoms that disrupt your ability to cope with life, report it to your doctor.

Premenstrual Dysphoric Disorder

A less common but even more severe type of premenstrual syndrome is premenstrual dysphoric disorder (PMDD). Women who suffer from PMDD often experience severe depression, anxiety, sleep disturbances, and fatigue in addition to a wide range of physical disturbances. The symptoms can be serious, and sometimes include suicidal thoughts. Women who have Seasonal Affective Disorder (SAD) usually have PMDD as well. Though PMS and PMDD differ in severity, diagnosis, and treatment, both seem to be linked to the way the body processes and responds to reproductive hormones.

Doctors diagnose PMS and PMDD based on when a woman's symptoms occur, not just the symptoms themselves. If you want to track your own premenstrual symptoms, you can keep a menstrual journal (see Appendix B: Keeping a Menopause Journal, for suggestions). If symptoms repeat at specific intervals, they may indicate PMS.

What Causes Menopause?

The average woman has about 400 reproductive cycles during her lifetime. As time goes on, the reproductive organs begin to respond to lowering hormone levels, causing periods to become first irregular, and then stop altogether. Every woman does this at her own rate, but the progression is somewhat predictable.

Follicles and Hormones

In every cycle, the woman's pituitary gland produces follicle-stimulating hormones (FSH) that trigger the follicle cells (small pouches) in the ovary that surround the developing eggs to produce estrogen, which in turn prepares an egg (usually just one) for fertilization. Each month, as the body's level of estrogen increases, the pituitary gland stops producing FSH and starts producing luteinizing hormone (LH), which causes the ovary to ovulate (release the egg) and produce progesterone, which in turn prepares the uterine lining to accept the fertilized egg.

The mature egg is only one of several "candidates" available each month. Those that don't mature (develop enough to be available for fertilization) are reabsorbed by the body. If the mature egg isn't fertilized, it, too, is reabsorbed and the lining of the uterus is shed during your period. The body's level of estrogen then dips, which triggers the FSH production that starts the whole cycle again.

"Running Out" of Eggs

Until recently it was thought that every woman was born with a set number of eggs, ranging from 400,000 to 700,000, and that half of those eggs deteriorated and were reabsorbed by each girl's body before she reaches puberty. Scientists are still researching whether this is accurate and how it works. Some new studies in mice suggest that there may be "germ cells" that develop into eggs throughout a woman's life. Whether these germ cells replenish your eggs or not, it does seem that over time your follicle cells stop responding to FSH, and you stop ovulating. As a result—over a period of years—you stop menstruating and your ovaries stop making estrogen and progesterone. You may continue to have menstrual periods after you stop ovulating, since your body continues to produce some estrogen. Most women notice a change in the frequency, duration, and flow of their periods during the three to four years before they stop menstruating completely. That's why you can't truly know that you've gone through menopause until a full twelve months have passed since your last period.

Taking a Closer Look at Perimenopause

Perimenopause, which means "around menopause," can last anywhere from two to ten years and usually begins sometime in a woman's mid- to late forties, and lasts until a year or so after the last period. Eventually, your ovaries completely stop all egg production and menstruation permanently ceases—that's menopause. Though perimenopause differs for every woman it generally marks a time of less-frequent ovulation and fluctuating levels of hormones, including estrogen, progesterone, and FSH.

 Fact

The term premenopause is no longer used to refer to the years preceding menopause, because all the years of a woman's life that precede menopause are premenopause. Today, "perimenopause" is used to describe the years when a woman's reproductive system slows down as it approaches menopause.

Your Very Own Trip

But knowing when and why you stop menstruating doesn't help you prepare to take an active part in managing your health through the perimenopause journey. In fact, it's more like being prepared for a trip to France knowing only your airport names and flight times. Hearing that you fly out of LaGuardia, spend five hours in the air, land at Charles de Gaulle airport, spend ten days in France, and then return to LaGuardia from Charles de Gaulle doesn't do much to help you plan a good trip. And the average statistics of the menopause journey don't tell you much either. Though no one can describe exactly what your experience in perimenopause and menopause will involve, some key bits of information about what others have experienced can help you prepare for the journey.

Orient Yourself for the Journey

The information in this chapter and the next is your perimenopause orientation session. Understanding what's ahead will help you feel more comfortable and relaxed when you experience menopause so that you're better able to pass smoothly through every stop along the way, ready and able to deal with any problems you may encounter.

Health Concerns

Women in the perimenopause period understandably become very aware of their health. Some of this awareness is from the symptoms they experience as their estrogen levels drop, and some arises from the health risks that occur after forty. Symptoms of perimenopause can be distressing and bothersome, but they are usually temporary and decrease over time, or can be treated. Genuine health risks that can cause chronic disease or serious illness must be detected and managed as soon as possible so that they do not shorten your life.

Common, but Manageable

The most common physical symptoms of the perimenopause are hot flashes, irregular and heavy menstrual periods, incontinence (leaking urine), heart palpitations, and weight gain. These are not only common but also usually treatable. Although not life threatening, they can impact your everyday life in significant ways. You may not die if you wet your pants, but you will probably be "embarrassed to death." When these symptoms begin to affect your quality of life, it is time to talk with your medical provider about how to deal with them.

More Serious Symptoms

Serious health issues may also arise at this time of your life. These are not just a nuisance, they can also lead to life-altering disability. Some of the most common serious conditions to be on the lookout for are high blood pressure, diabetes, heart disease, cancer, arthritis, and osteoporosis. It is easy to dismiss early signs of these conditions as just "aches and pains of old age." But paying attention early on can save you a lot of discomfort and even save your life.

If you notice that there is a significant change in any area of your physical ability, check it out with your provider. Be on the lookout for these symptoms:

- Shortness of breath
- Losing or gaining weight although you haven't changed your eating patterns
- Inability to move as easily as you used to
- Feeling extremely tired
- Inability to walk or stand as much as you could a year ago
- Thirst and needing to urinate frequently

If you suffer from any of these symptoms, be sure to talk to your medical professional. These are all signs that something serious could be going on, and the earlier you know the sooner you can do something about it. Continue to have pap smears and mammograms. Get a colonoscopy at fifty to rule out and prevent future colon cancers. Have your health provider listen to your heart and lungs. Get your blood pressure taken and your blood work checked. Any and all of these can help you head off serious illness.

 Alert

> If you have a sudden onset of extreme symptoms—such as severe headaches, extremely heavy bleeding, chest pain, difficulty breathing, severe fatigue, and unusual bloating or weight loss—see your health care provider. Severe, sudden, or long-lasting symptoms may be related to some serious illness or disease. You need to report them right away.

Emotional Concerns

Many women (or their partners) say that they become "more emotional" as menopause approaches. As hormone levels drop, and particularly if you are someone who suffers marked emotional changes premenstrually, you may notice that you don't seem to have the same control over your emotions as you used to. This may be a temporary response to physiologic changes, or it may be the sign of serious mental health concerns. It's worth a discussion with your health provider to sort that out. If your provider is someone who sees lots of perimenopausal women, he or she has a broad experience with the range of symptoms around menopause. You may need some help deciding whether you are "going crazy" or just passing through perimenopause.

At the same time that your hormones are fluctuating, you may also be going through truly trying emotional times. Losses such as children moving out, parents ill or dying, divorce, or job changes can overwhelm your ability to cope. Grief and depression may interfere with your day-to-day life and need to be addressed. If you have a family history of depression, or have struggled with it in the past, stay alert to the possibility that you could become clinically depressed and might need treatment.

Serious or Not?

Some of the symptoms of fluctuating hormones can be mistaken for, or can trigger, more serious mental health issues. Occasional anxiety is not the same as panic disorder; having a "blue" afternoon is not as ominous as having suicidal thoughts; irritability can be a normal variation, while rage is not. Sometimes it is difficult to sort through your experience of these emotional changes without professional help.

Grieving Your Youth

Another loss that women feel at this time and may be reluctant to discuss is the loss of their youth. As your children become more adult and involved in their own lives, and as you see the early signs of aging in your face and body, you begin to realize that you are no longer a youngster. In a culture where youth is valued (worshipped!), it is easy to think of yourself as less valuable. If you were always appreciated for your looks, you may feel a loss of power over your life. If your energy is beginning to lessen, you may think you are losing your ability to compete. Even though you may feel more confident in your life, you may still feel the loss of your youth, and that can provoke sadness, grief, and even depression.

☐ Essential

Don't confuse depression—feelings of despair, hopelessness, lack of energy, and a diluted interest in life around you—with mood swings. When feelings of despair last more than a few weeks, you should consult your doctor. Untreated depression can damage your life and future.

Social and Family Concerns

Midlife is a time of family and social upheaval for many women. There are many aspects of life that shift or change as you go through your forties and fifties. Your marriage, your children, your parents, your job situation, and your peer group can all present challenges.

Your Marriage

Midlife can bring many changes to your marriage or relationship. Even if you have been together for many years, you may discover that busy lives and separate jobs have made you strangers to each other. While many couples look forward to an "empty nest" in order to enjoy the peace and privacy of being a couple again, others find that they are uncomfortable spending more time together. It is a time for reassessment of life priorities and can be very unsettling as people define their future together. If your relationship has been rocky in the past but children or careers distracted you from seeing the flaws, midlife can be an uncomfortable awakening. And if you have longed for more time together, it can be a second honeymoon. Like everything about the menopause journey, it is highly individual and there are lots of opportunities for reinventing your life and love relationships.

Your Children

If you have children, they are getting older, too. They may be leaving for school or work, and slipping out from your watchful eye and protection. The range in your children's ages can be anything from toddlers to independent adults as you go through this passage of menopause. Obviously, this can be the source of both worry and delight. You may be anxious about the money to put your kids through college, or worried about how to get services for a special needs child or grandchild. You may have grown children living with you who want their own freedom and control over their lives but don't yet have the means to live on their own. Your energy may be fading and you may not enjoy the conflict that raising teenagers can sometimes provoke. If your job has become increasingly responsible, you may have less time to spend at home, managing the needs of your children.

Sometimes this can be the perfect moment to begin teaching your children the skills of independence. But if you are still responsible for children of any age, it will take time and energy. Find resources to support you with your parenting. Extended family, social services, local children's hospitals, company employee-assistance programs, and friends can all offer suggestions for whatever type of parenting support you might need.

Your Friends

Many women consider friends to be their lifesavers in times of turmoil. If you have friends who are in the perimenopausal years, they will relate to your experience and be your companions on the road. Younger and older friends, too, can enrich your life and offer you perspective. Tell your friends what your menopausal experience is like for you. Help them understand the changes, and let them support you when you need a little boost.

Find friends who are positive and helpful. If you are feeling sad or irritable, work with your friends to find ways to make sure that your mood won't damage your friendships. A sense of humor shared with a friend can see you through tough times. Cranky teenagers and aging parents are all handled better if you have a friend to confide in.

L. Essential

Being a caretaker is hard work—don't go it alone. If you are responsible for an aging parent, you will need support. The U.S. Department of Health and Human Services has an Eldercare Locator that can help you explore the services available in the area where your parent lives. You can contact them at *www.eldercare.gov/Eldercare/Public/Home.asp* or by calling their toll-free number at 800-677-1116.

Your Parents

They don't call this life stage the "sandwich generation" for nothing. It is very common for people of this age to be parenting their own children while becoming increasingly responsible for aging or fragile parents. If your parent lives nearby, you may become their caretaker, and if they live far away, you may find yourself worrying about their health and well-being. This is not an easy or simple responsibility, and it may take family time and resources to support them in their later years.

As with other relationships, this is a time of life to find a comfortable place emotionally with your parents. The time spent with them can be a source of memory building and friendship. You will be trying to respect their need for autonomy and still protect them from hazards such as falling and disease. Although the role reversal can be trying, it is also a chance to rework your connection as adults. Most importantly, keep yourself healthy within it. Make use of any informal and professional supports available to you to preserve your health and sanity. Set up Meals on Wheels for your widowed father. Get your mother's weekly grocery list, and arrange for delivery via Internet if it is available in her town. Take it on as a family project, if your family is able, and have your teenagers spend time doing errands for their grandparents. Sit down with your family and let them help you think about ways to assist your parents respectfully in their time of failing health. Your family may surprise you with their creative suggestions for dealing with grandma or grandpa. And you are modeling for your children how to cope with the situation. Someday they may be in your shoes, helping *you* make decisions. Show them how it can be done.

CHAPTER 4

Perimenopause— Adjusting to the Changes

LIKE ADOLESCENCE, perimenopause is full of surprises for you and your body. Suddenly your physical responses are unpredictable, and it can be a little unnerving. Your adolescence was marked by a growth spurt, new ways of thinking, sudden emotional responses, and a body becoming sexual in appearance and sensations. Now hot flashes, sudden emotional responses, and a body changing in its appearance and sexual response mark your menopause. This chapter will familiarize you with common menopausal symptoms, and later chapters will offer ways of dealing with these changes.

The Journey Through Perimenopause

Every individual menopause, like every adolescence, is its own story. On average, women begin perimenopause at age forty-seven and experience it for about four years. But women can enter perimenopause in their late thirties or early fifties, and it can last from a few months to eight or ten years. You have no way of knowing precisely when or how you'll begin noticing the changes that announce your coming menopause. Instead, you're more likely to find yourself one day connecting the dots of a number of odd symptoms and changes that eventually add up to the fact that you are, indeed, moving toward menopause.

Whew, It's Just Menopause!

Whenever it happens, you're likely to have a difficult time accepting the idea that you actually are perimenopausal, but the realization can be a relief. You may have decided that you were losing your mind or developing an odd and difficult-to-diagnose illness, when in reality the symptoms you experience are normal, manageable demonstrations of a natural stage in your body's development.

Uh-oh, It's Menopause!

The opposite reaction is also common. Once you realize that you are not coming down with a tropical fever or going over the edge with a mental disorder, you may find yourself worried or fearful that you are entering a scary, unknown land of hot flashes and brittle bones. This book should help you sort out what is normal and expected. The more you know about the possibilities, the better you can cope with them. And just as with adolescence, a list of "typical" symptoms will only give you some ideas about what might happen. Your own passage will be unique to you, and you will be the one to decide when you need support to deal with the changes, and which ones you can ride out on your own.

Recognizing the Symptoms

So what can a woman expect from perimenopause? What kinds of symptoms are common—or even possible—and what do they mean? If you have to listen to your body in order to understand its condition and needs, how do you interpret the messages of perimenopausal symptoms? And how do you know if your symptoms are related to perimenopause or some other part of the aging process?

You Are the Expert on What's Normal for You

First, it's important to understand that, if you think it may be perimenopause, it probably is. No one is more familiar than you are with your body's feelings and reactions during your monthly cycles. As the following sections demonstrate, women have reported a wide variety of symptoms during and after perimenopause. Remember, some women experience no symptoms at all.

It's also important to keep in mind that everyone can expect to experience some physical and mental signs of aging. As women age, many of their physical changes are triggered or exacerbated by hormonal fluctuations. The good news is, any overt symptom that is associated with changing hormone levels can be temporary—and may even be diminished through diet, exercise, or other healthy options.

Perimenopause isn't like measles; you don't wake up one day with a clear sign that you've come down with a case of waning estrogen. So identifying when you enter perimenopause isn't always easy. If you start noticing obvious changes in the length of your periods, the intervals between them, or the heaviness of your flow, and you're between the ages of thirty-five and sixty, you should start checking for other signs of perimenopause.

 ## Fact

Don't let the term "symptoms" lead you to believe that this chapter is describing perimenopause as a disease or illness—it's neither. Perimenopause is a natural process of physical change. For the sake of simplicity, this book refers to the body's demonstrations of this natural process as "symptoms," with no connotation of illness or disease.

Other Early Changes

Changes in your cycle may not be your first indicator that perimenopause is approaching. Many women report symptoms of perimenopause while their periods remain much the same. Most women feel some or all of the following symptoms as their bodies prepare to stop ovulating:

- Hot flashes
- Mood swings
- Decreased sexual drive
- Weight gain
- Difficulty concentrating
- Heart palpitations
- Migraine headaches
- Irregular and/or heavy periods
- Involuntary urine release and bladder urgency
- Insomnia
- Vaginal dryness and painful intercourse
- Anxiety or panic attacks

Add to that list everything from aching joints and muscles to the onset of chin whiskers and you've still only started to talk about the wide variety of symptoms perimenopausal women have reported. Though some women report no symptoms of approaching menopause, most women do experience symptoms so chances are good that you will too. Thinning hair, hot flashes, aching joints—these and other symptoms may seem like inevitable side effects of the aging process. But many symptoms of the aging processes can be triggered or exaggerated by the hormonal fluctuations of perimenopause.

If the preceding list paints a scary picture of perimenopause, it's also important to mention that even among women who experience one or more of these symptoms, their effects can be mild, transient, or otherwise bearable. Your body is adjusting to varying rates of hormones during perimenopause; the signs and symptoms of that adjustment are often temporary and disappear after your body has acclimated itself to its new hormone levels. The following sections offer you a closer look at these symptoms so that you have a better idea of what to expect.

Essential

Don't dismiss symptoms or make up your mind that you're going to tough it out no matter what. You have options for alleviating symptoms—lifestyle changes, behavior modification, hormone therapy, or dietary changes. Do yourself a favor and explore your options

Physical Changes

Your body will tell you when you are entering perimenopause. You may not listen to it at first, or you may try to dismiss physical symptoms as "getting a bug" or some other familiar event. But once it gets your attention, you can tune in to your body and manage some of the physical changes before they get the best of you. Here are some common changes to watch for.

Hot Flashes (Including Night Sweats)

Along with irregularities in menses, hot flashes have to earn the dubious honor of being one of the symptoms most commonly reported by women during perimenopause. Nearly 75 percent of women who report perimenopausal symptoms list hot flashes among them. Hot flashes can come at any time of the day or night, but when they occur during sleep, they're usually referred to as night sweats.

Hot flashes can be mild or severe, but in general, they involve a fast-spreading sensation of warmth in your neck, shoulders, and face that may last a few seconds or as long as thirty minutes or more. This sensation may begin at the top of your scalp, behind your ears, on your chest, or even across your nose. Hot flashes don't have to limit themselves to your head and shoulders; many women have also reported flashes occurring across the breasts, below the breasts, or all over the body. Hot flashes are so common and bothersome that Chapter 5 is devoted entirely to managing them.

Irregular and/or Heavy Periods

Changes in your period are usually the very first sign that the perimenopause has arrived. Even if your periods have always been as regular as clockwork, you can expect some irregularities to occur in the years preceding menopause. The levels of estrogen and progesterone produced in your body can flag and surge, contributing to unusually light or skipped periods, or periods that flow for weeks at a time. Some women experience spotting—or even phases of heavy bleeding—for a few days between periods. In other words, you may find that irregularity becomes the norm in your perimenopausal cycles.

 Alert

If periods come less than twenty-one days apart, last more than a week, are unusually heavy, and maintain these irregularities for more than two cycles, make an appointment with your doctor or health care professional for a gynecological checkup.

Having said that heavy periods and ongoing irregular bleeding are not uncommon during perimenopause, it's also important to have them checked out by your health care provider. Heavy bleeding or bleeding that continues for a long time can be more than an inconvenience. Non-stop heavy bleeding can leave you tired, weak, and anemic—a prime candidate for getting a cold, flu, or infections. Even more importantly, heavy bleeding may have nothing to do with simple hormonal ebbs and flows. Heavy bleeding could be a sign of abnormal tissue in the uterus, precancerous conditions, or even endometrial cancer. Don't take chances that your period irregularities are just part of the change. If your irregularities are dramatic, see your health care professional. (For complications of the uterus and their treatment, see Chapter 6.)

 Fact

According to some studies, your menstrual cycles may shorten before age forty, then lengthen slightly as you approach menopause. So while your period may occur every twenty-six days when you're forty years old, as you reach forty-five, thirty-five-day cycles may be normal for you.

Heart Palpitations

Heart palpitations are the sudden uncomfortable awareness that your heart is pounding, often at a more rapid rate than normal. Heart palpitations can be frightening, but remember that they aren't uncommon in perimenopausal and menopausal women. Certainly, these women aren't the only ones to experience palpitations—many men and women have them after exercising, when frightened, or while taking some medications. But at menopause, the incidence of heart palpitations seems to rise in women.

Women describe heart palpitations differently, but in general a heart palpitation feels like your heart is beating rapidly, out of sequence, too strenuously, or in some other abnormal fashion. A heart palpitation can feel like no more than a brief fluttering in your chest that passes within a matter of a few seconds. Other, stronger palpitations can feel like a distinct pounding in your chest that lasts a few minutes and can leave you feeling light-headed or short of breath.

Essential

Caffeine, cigarettes, and excess sugar can overstimulate your system and be a contributing factor in heart palpitations. Perimenopause is a great time to cut back on your intake of these.

Involuntary Urine Release

If you've ever experienced urinary tract infections (UTI), you might feel as though they're back with a vengeance during your transition into menopause. And if you've never had urinary tract problems, you might develop them during perimenopause. According to some estimates, nearly 20 percent of all women over the age of forty-five develop some urinary tract problems. Those problems can include UTIs, stress urinary incontinence (caused by a stressor such as sneezing, coughing, or laughing), and urge incontinence (caused by a bladder spasm that forces urine out, even when the bladder is not completely full).

Weight Gain

The results are in: weight gain is commonly seen as people of both sexes age. The term "middle age spread" was coined decades ago to describe the tendency of the post-forty body to take on excess weight. Of course, not everyone gains weight during perimenopause and after menopause, and not everyone who does gain weight gains debilitating amounts. But the fact is that the majority of women report weight gain at this time. Even women who don't gain weight may experience a change in their body shape. Many women in middle age gain softer, rounder abdomens, larger hips, thicker waistlines, and even extra weight on their shoulders, arms, and thighs.

Neurological and Cognitive Changes

As your hormone levels change, your brain function may show signs of faltering. This can be a frustrating and unsettling side effect of the menopausal process, and sometimes it's best to relax and realize it can also be normal.

Difficulty Concentrating

If you're approaching fifty, and it seems as though you aren't quite as sharp mentally as you used to be, it's probably because you aren't. Though fuzzy thinking, forgetfulness, difficulty concentrating, and memory problems are common complaints of perimenopausal and menopausal women, these issues are linked as closely with the aging process as they are to changing ovarian functions. Today, doctors and health care professionals recognize that certain cognitive problems are due to depleted estrogen levels and other changes in the aging brain.

How does this fuzzy thinking manifest itself? In ways you've probably experienced most of your life, for example, losing your car keys, forgetting what you were about to say, recognizing a face but failing to recall the name, searching fruitlessly for the right word, being easily distracted, or losing your train of thought. As women reach the age of menopause (around age fifty), however, they can suffer an increase in these sorts of problems. You may have heard people refer to these lapses as "senior moments," and if you're approaching the age of menopause you're likely to be experiencing them yourself.

While you can't stop your brain's odometer from registering the passing years, you can slow down and repair many of the issues that contribute to fuzzy thinking and other cognitive roadblocks. See Chapter 7 for more information.

Memory Loss

As your estrogen rises and falls during perimenopause, memory may be impacted. This is usually transitory and will improve once the body adjusts to new lower levels of hormones. It is a symptom that women can find annoying, or even alarming, if they are worried about dementia. Although some memory loss is very common with aging, especially short-term memory, these initial memory lapses should not be a cause for alarm unless they are serious enough to affect day-to-day activities. Stress can make memory problems worse, so take that into account when you are assessing whether this is a problem for you.

 Alert

> If your heart palpitations are severe or produce significant discomfort or side effects, you need to talk to your doctor or health care provider about them. Some palpitations are a warning sign of an impending heart attack. Pay attention to the number and frequency of your palpitations, and be prepared to discuss these and your heart history when you talk with your doctor.

Insomnia

Interruptions in normal sleep patterns are common complaints of perimenopausal and postmenopausal women. During the years approaching menopause, many women find that they wake once or twice during the night and then have a difficult time returning to sleep. Other times, women find that it takes longer for them to fall asleep when they go to bed at night or that they awaken an hour or two earlier than they used to. Whatever form it takes, insomnia leaves women feeling tired, irritable, and out of touch with their surroundings.

Fortunately, many women find that insomnia is a transient problem that may last no more than a few months. For others, insomnia during perimenopause may be so severe that it hampers their performance and sense of well-being during the day. Chapter 7 offers a number of options for minimizing insomnia when it strikes. As always, if your symptoms become severe, consult your doctor or health care professional. You can combat insomnia, so don't allow it to drag you down during this important transition phase.

Migraines and Other Headaches

Some medical experts will tell you that migraine headaches aren't truly a symptom of menopause. Nevertheless, many women who have never experienced a migraine in their lives begin having them during perimenopause. These hormonally related migraines are often experienced by younger women in the first few days of their periods, or during pregnancy. In both cases, fluctuations in your body's estrogen levels seem to be a cause.

Though both sexes suffer from migraines, women are three times more likely to have them. Migraines are intensely painful headaches thought to be associated with constricted blood vessels in the brain. Women who suffer migraines describe them as pounding headaches that can cause nausea, vomiting, and a strong sensitivity to light, noise, and odors. Some migraine sufferers—about twenty percent—report a certain premonition, or aura, for several minutes before the actual pain begins. This aura can include flashing lights, certain odors, changes in their vision, or numbness in a hand, arm, or leg. Migraines usually last four or more hours, and they can last as long as a week.

Migraines aren't the only kind of headaches that seem to accompany perimenopause. In general, women report having more frequent and severe headaches during this time. These are usually simple stress or muscle tension headaches, and are often relieved by over-the-counter analgesics such as aspirin and acetaminophen.

Emotional and Psychological Changes

Women report various emotional and psychological shifts during perimenopause. Sometimes their partners or families complain about this symptom. As with other perimenopausal symptoms, these changes can be temporary, but they can also be unnerving.

Mood Swings

The good news about mood swings is that you may never experience them during perimenopause. Still, mood swings are a common complaint of perimenopausal women, and among women who cite symptoms in perimenopause, nearly 50 percent say mood swings are among the symptoms that bother them the most.

Whether you think of them as moodiness, temporary depression, or simply the blues, mood swings can be minor "speed bumps" in your day—or they can leave you feeling totally down and out. The experiences are as individual as the women who have them, but mood swings tend to take the form of intensified emotional reactions. Sometimes, the swing can take you high, and you feel a particularly strong delight in everything around you—the weather, a movie, your dinner companion. Other times, however, mood swings can take you on a wild roller-coaster ride of emotions, such as intense sorrow, despair, love, anger, anxiety, general depression, or fear. A typical anger response during a mood swing can leave your heart pounding, your face flushed, and your head throbbing. Mood swings can trigger bouts of crying and cause deep, dark feelings of hopelessness. Then, however dramatic they might be, mood swings may pass rather quickly, leaving you feeling a bit shaken and confused by the emotional ride.

 Alert

> Although it is tempting to drink alcohol when feeling anxious, it is a very bad idea for menopausal women. Not only does it cause insomnia and trigger hot flashes, according to the North American Menopause Society, women who drink heavily have a higher death rate from alcohol abuse, and are at a higher risk for stroke, liver disease, and cancer.

Though mood swings seem to be emotional responses, they can, in fact, be a direct physical response to the changing hormonal levels in your bloodstream. In fact, many perimenopausal women experience mood swings along with other common symptoms of premenstrual syndrome (PMS), even when those women have never before suffered from PMS symptoms. Those symptoms include a wide range of physical and emotional markers, including gastrointestinal distress, headaches, pains in muscles and joints, fatigue, heart pounding, hot flashes, exaggerated sensitivity to sounds and smells, agitation, and insomnia.

Depression
Depression is a serious condition that should not be confused with brief episodes of feeling sad or overwhelmed. It is not a normal part

of perimenopause, although many women use "depressed" to describe their quickly changing moods or tendency to cry easily. Chapter 8 discusses depression and its treatment in greater detail. If you find yourself feeling hopeless, desperate, or sad for long periods of time, see your health care provider or counselor to determine if this is part of adjusting to new hormone levels or something more serious.

 Fact

Most health care professionals agree that certain lifestyle habits contribute to insomnia at any time in your life. Get regular exercise and try not to consume any alcohol, sugar, caffeine, or rich foods within the two to three hours before bedtime.

Changes in Libido

Few things are more individual than libido. Everyone has a unique attitude toward sex and sexuality, and we all differ in our sexual habits and desires. While this undeniable (and delightful!) individuality may seem to contradict any generalizations about how sexual desire can change during menopause, many women do experience some types of changes during this time.

Many studies—including those of the famous Alfred Kinsey—indicate that both men and women can experience gradually declining sexual desire as they age. Pay special attention to the "can" in that last sentence. While not everyone undergoes a noticeable change in libido during menopause, many women report changes in their level of sexual desire. Some say they have more interest in sex and enjoy it more, while others say their desires have diminished, and still others say they find sex increasingly unappealing—even painful.

Other Perimenopausal Changes You May Notice

Recognizing the unique experience each of us has as we age, most of us can expect to experience other physical changes during—and perhaps as a result of—the physical changes of perimenopause. If perimenopause occurs during a woman's forties, for example, here are some of the changes her body might be undergoing:

- Muscles may lose mass more easily and become harder to tone during your forties, so your old workout plan may not be enough to maintain the strength and body weight you enjoyed in your thirties. You may need a new workout program during this time; see Chapter 17.
- Bones can start to lose calcium as estrogen levels recede and the body becomes less efficient at absorbing calcium from food. You may need to adjust your diet to include more vitamin D and calcium, or consider taking supplements. See Chapter 15 for more information.
- Eyes become less efficient as the lenses lose elasticity and their controlling muscles weaken, making focusing close-up more difficult. Estrogen helps keep eyes and muscles elastic, so diminishing levels of estrogen contribute to this degeneration.
- Skin and hair can begin to thin in response to lowered levels of estrogen; most people start to get some gray hair in their forties. Estrogen also helps maintain the collagen content (the basic protein bridgework) of your skin, thus keeping it youthful and elastic. Your strong ally in the battle against this aging factor is a healthy diet and lots and lots of water. See Chapter 16 for more information.
- Metabolism slows down during your forties, so weight gain can creep up on you. Typical dieting methods are unlikely to work as well for you at this age, so maintaining or losing weight may require additional exercise and calorie cutting.
- Propensities for certain conditions such as diabetes and asthma can accelerate during this time, due to changing hormone levels, lowered resistance to stress and infections, and other factors of aging. Medical checkups and health maintenance are more essential than ever at this point.

Don't be put off by this list; yes, the perimenopause may be an introduction to the beginning of the aging process and the toll it takes on your body's systems. But there's never been a time when medicine and health care, public information, and healthy life practices have been better able to contribute to everyone's pursuit of a healthy, active middle age. You have more control than any generation that's preceded you in how quickly or slowly your body loses ground to the aging process. You can learn ways to manage the effects of perimenopause and its role in the aging process.

Essential

If you've been casual about your health until you hit forty (which most people are), now is a perfect time to get serious about preparing for a long, healthy life ahead. Diet, exercise, lifestyle changes, and regular medical checkups are your strongest agents for maintaining a strong, healthy body.

Stay on Top of Your Symptoms

This chapter has outlined a wide range of symptoms that can appear during the years preceding menopause. But it's important to remember that you may experience none, some, or all of these symptoms—or others that aren't even listed. To be certain that you are doing all you can to maintain peak health during this important time of transition, pay close attention to your body, and don't ignore the messages it sends you. Many of the symptoms that initially seem par for the course for middle age may be symptoms of problems requiring serious and quick medical treatment. So don't ignore any ongoing problem because you think it's just "the change." Work closely with your health care provider to make sure that your body gets any and all of the help that it needs to stay strong, fit, and healthy.

Chapter 5

Coping with Hot Flashes

WHEN WOMEN TALK about the bothersome aspects of menopause, hot flashes are the symptom they cite—and complain about—most often. Though hot flashes fade over time, severe symptoms can disrupt both the waking and sleeping hours of your busy life for several years. Fortunately, there are many ways to relieve or reduce hot flashes, but you need to choose carefully—and be sure to consult with your health care professional.

Hot Flash Facts

Hot flashes are considered a "vasomotor" symptom. This means they are the result of a change in your body's ability to regulate the opening and closing of blood vessels. About 75 percent of all women passing through the stages of menopause will experience hot flashes during some part of the transition. Though hot flashes are a common symptom of menopause, in many cases they are a minor inconvenience rather than an alarming problem. Hot flashes (sometimes called hot flushes) often begin with an increase in heart rate and a slight feeling of warmth, usually occurring in the face, neck, and shoulders.

A Range of Symptoms

Women describe hot flashes differently, depending upon how frequent or how dramatic their symptoms are. Mild or moderate hot flashes may last anywhere from one to fifteen minutes and cause feelings of mild warmth, accompanied by light perspiration and a slightly dry mouth. After the flash passes, the skin may feel slightly clammy. Mild hot flashes pass with little or no impact on general feelings of well-being.

Severe hot flashes can last from thirty seconds to thirty minutes and cause the skin temperature to rise dramatically. The face, neck, and throat can become flushed and red, and the body can break out in heavy perspiration. A woman experiencing a severe hot flash can have difficulty breathing, and the hot flash can trigger panic attacks and anxiety. Afterward, the woman may be left with a headache, some nausea, and a general feeling of anxiety and exhaustion.

If hot flashes are severe or long lasting, they can have a negative impact on your health and well-being. Hot flashes that occur at night—often known as night sweats—can interrupt sleep and lead to daytime fatigue, exhaustion, and decreased mental abilities. The fear of breaking into a clothes-drenching sweat at work or during social events can lead to anxiety and even depression. When hot flashes ruin your sleep or prevent you from performing well during the day, it's time to take action.

What's Happening When You Have a Hot Flash?

Hot flashes are connected to changes in your estrogen levels, though the specific cause and effect relationship is still under study. Recent studies seem to point to a narrower "thermoneutral zone" in some women, meaning that their range of comfortable temperature becomes narrower. It is a lowering of the "sweat threshold" and your body is prompted to sweat with even small rises in body temperature.

Declining levels of estrogen set the stage for hot flashes and the actual hot flashes are the result of this sudden resetting of the body's thermostat. If your brain senses that your body is even a bit too hot—for any reason, including increased blood flow to the brain, a high ambient temperature, or even the ingestion of hot, spicy foods—it sends out a signal that your body needs to cool off, now! In response, your pituitary gland sends out luteinizing hormone (LH), which causes the blood vessels near your skin's surface to dilate to release heat through your skin. This heat-releasing action makes your skin temperature (and your body temperature) rise, followed by an increase in perspiration. The perspiration helps to cool the skin, which can result in a clammy feeling. If you've perspired heavily, you may be left damp and even chilly. Your body temperature drops and your blood vessels constrict. If you are damp and cold, you may begin to shiver. That's the hot flash in action.

Common Hot Flash Triggers

Estrogen levels alone do not predict hot flashes and other factors can cause them or contribute to their severity. Many women find, for example, that they have hot flashes during periods of anxiety and nervousness; other studies have found that some prescription blood pressure medications and anti-anxiety medications may also cause hot flashes. Hot flashes may be your body's reaction to certain foods or beverages or even the temperature of the air around you—some women report their hot flashes are more severe and last longer when they occur during hot weather or in a hot room.

 Alert

If you suffer from severe hot flashes, it's not unusual to have feelings of nausea, headache, and weakness afterward—especially when hot flashes last for more than fifteen minutes. If your feelings of intense heat last for longer than an hour, it may be something more serious, and you should tell your doctor or other health care professional.

How Many, How Bad, How Long?

Although many women don't seem to notice hot flashes until after menopause has occurred, many others begin having them during perimenopause, with forty-eight being an average age for the onset of hot flashes. In general, women who experience hot flashes start having them at least one year before menopause, and continue having them for one to six years.

The American College of Obstetricians and Gynecologists's publication *Managing Menopause* lists the findings of one study in which 501 women were asked about the frequency and severity of their hot flashes. Of those participating in the study, 87 percent reported having one or more flashes per day; of those experiencing multiple daily hot flashes, the numbers of incidents per day ranged from five to fifty, with one-third of the women reporting more than ten. Another study reported a lower frequency of hot flashes—participants had an average of only three or four flashes a day.

Techniques for Turning Down the Heat

A number of treatment options to help you lessen—or even eliminate—hot flashes caused by the onset of menopause are discussed later in this chapter. But you have a variety of first-defense techniques available to you that don't require any special medication or therapeutic program.

Start with the Obvious

When you first begin to notice that hot flashes are part of your life, you can try to diminish them. Try these simple techniques to avoid hot flashes or minimize their severity:

- **Avoid triggering foods and drinks.** Spicy foods—foods heavy in capsaicin, the heat-inducing chemical in cayenne and other hot peppers—can trigger hot flashes. Caffeine and alcohol are also common triggers.
- **Drink plenty of water during the day—at least thirty-two ounces, more if possible.** Keep a glass of ice water with you at work and during meetings and set a thermal-lined drink container of ice water on your nightstand, ready to help cool down raging flashes.
- **Get at least thirty minutes of exercise every day.** Exercise, including stretching, aerobic, and weight-bearing activities, has been shown to cut down on the frequency of hot flashes, and may even help limit their length and severity.
- **Wear layers of moisture-absorbing clothing.** When a hot flash strikes, you can take off one or more layers of clothing to help cool your skin temperature quickly. Cotton fabrics are particularly helpful in allowing adequate air to reach the skin, and they're good at absorbing perspiration.
- **Keep your thermostat turned down—seventy degrees or lower during the day, and sixty-five degrees or lower at night.** Lower temperatures can help ward off hot flashes.

- **Manage stress to the best of your ability.** Avoid stress if you can, but be prepared for stressful situations you can't sidestep. Deep breathing exercises, meditation, yoga, and visualization are all helpful techniques for boosting your ability to remain calm and centered throughout your day.

L, Essential

If a hot flash strikes, you may get some quick relief by running cold water over your hands, wrists, and inner elbow. A cold cloth on your forehead or the back of your neck can help, too; if you're at home, step into a cold shower and let the water run over you until the heat wave passes.

Don't Be Discouraged

If you take all the steps listed above, and still find yourself doused in sweat several times a day, don't despair. Continue to do the common sense things that will reduce hot flashes, but also consider talking to your health care provider about what other treatments might work. You will be able to say that you've tried the simple things, and your symptoms are serious enough that you need something more. And remember that sometimes tricks that don't work one day are magic the next. Finding the combination that works for you is as much art as science.

Hormonal Treatments for Hot Flash Relief

Though medical science continues to study the connection between hormone depletion and hot flashes, hormone therapy—involving estrogen and/or progesterone—is the most effective medical treatment for vasomotor symptoms known today. According to the American College of Obstetricians and Gynecologists, 80 to 90 percent of women taking prescribed estrogen find relief from hot flashes.

Estrogen Therapy

While it's true that estrogen offers a number of other health benefits for women experiencing symptoms of perimenopause and menopause, including protection against osteoporosis and colorectal cancer, there are also risks in using it. It is not as commonly prescribed as it was in years past, and may be seen as a second choice solution, after you have tried some of the nonhormonal remedies. You and your health care provider can decide if your menopausal symptoms, including hot flashes, are worth the risk of using estrogen therapy. Your personal and family health history can help you make a decision about using hormone therapy, and your health provider can help you sort it all out.

Estrogen is not recommended for women with a personal history of recently diagnosed endometrial cancer. For these women, progestins—such as medroxyprogesterone or megestrol acetate—have been shown to offer relief from hot flashes. Some studies have shown progestins to decrease hot flashes by as much as 70 to 90 percent.

 Fact

Estrogen is a highly effective tool for combating symptoms of perimenopause and menopause, but it's not suitable for all women. See Chapter 11 for more information about the benefits and potential risks of hormone therapies.

Progesterone Therapy

Another hormone-based treatment for hot flashes is progesterone cream. This cream, available by prescription, is rubbed on the skin, and the progesterone is slowly absorbed into the woman's system. Though some studies have shown that progesterone cream can offer significant relief from hot flashes, it can be accompanied by some negative side effects, including vaginal bleeding and PMS symptoms.

Again, your doctor or health care professional can help you decide whether or not hormone-based treatments are your best choice for reducing or eliminating hot flashes. If together you decide that hormones aren't right for you, you can choose from other treatment options, including other medications and hormone alternatives, discussed in the sections that follow.

Nonhormonal Medications

Though some medical experts readily prescribe some form of hormone therapy for the relief of vasomotor symptoms, these treatments aren't appropriate for all women. Women with active endometrial or breast cancers, for example, usually must avoid hormone therapy during cancer treatment. Medical professionals rarely prescribe hormone therapy for women with a personal or family history of blood clotting, liver disease, or other conditions that can be triggered or exacerbated by hormone treatments.

Medications That Can Help

To provide relief from hot flashes for women who cannot take estrogen, medical professionals can prescribe other medications that have been shown to offer some relief from hot flashes. The following list mentions some of these prescription medications for alleviating hot flashes:

- Clonidine hydrochloride reduces the responsiveness of the body's vascular system, and has been used for some time in the treatment of high blood pressure. A low dose is used and it may take three to four weeks to begin to see improvement in symptoms; blood pressure must also be monitored. Clonidine does have some negative side effects and can disrupt the sleep of some women. Other side effects reported include dizziness and dry mouth.
- Methyldopa is another antihypertensive (high blood pressure medication) sometimes used to relieve vasomotor symptoms. Though methyldopa has been shown to reduce the number of hot flashes women experience during the day, it can cause dry mouth, dizziness, and headaches.
- Selective serotonin reuptake inhibitors (SSRIs), including paroxetine, fluoxetine, and venlafaxine, are also used to lessen vasomotor symptoms, although they are not approved by the

Food and Drug Administration (FDA) for that purpose. In higher doses, these drugs are used to treat depression. Some tests have shown that relatively low doses of these drugs can reduce the frequency and severity of hot flashes anywhere from 19 to 60 percent, depending upon the specific drug and dosage strategy. Side effects of these drugs include dry mouth, nausea, and anxiety.

- Bellergal, a drug that combines very low dosages of belladonna and phenobarbital, is an FDA-approved medication for the treatment of menopausal symptoms. This drug has been used for decades in the short-term treatment of hot flashes, with varying success. Bellergal can have a number of unpleasant side effects, including constipation, dry mouth, and dizziness.

- Gabapentin is an anti-seizure medication that is sometimes prescribed for the treatment of hot flashes. In studies, 70 percent of women reported that they had a noticeable improvement in their symptoms. The long-term effects are not yet known, but one study showed gabapentin to be as effective as estrogen in reducing hot flashes, when compared to placebo. Side effects, which are lower if the medication is taken with meals, may include fatigue, dizziness, swelling of hands and feet, and skin rash.

 Alert

Many of the nonhormonal treatments for hot flashes and other menopause symptoms are controversial, and their effectiveness, safety, and possible side effects and interactions with other medications remain the subject of ongoing studies.

What's Best for You?

If hot flashes are making your life miserable, there are treatments that can help. You have to decide whether your symptoms are serious enough to need medical intervention and prescription medications. Short-term treatment for the relief of hot flashes is very common, but your own unique risks and family history need to be considered. Be honest with your care provider about the severity of your hot flashes so that together you can decide what, if any, medication would work best for you. If you think you'd like to try some non-prescription medications to treat your symptoms, ask your health care provider for suggestions. The following section discusses some of the common ones.

Herbs, Botanicals, and Other Alternatives

It's important to approach any alternative treatment option with open eyes and healthy skepticism. Botanical extracts, herbal supplements, and nutraceutical compounds aren't inspected or approved by the FDA, so they haven't passed the rigorous testing process of prescription medications, and they haven't undergone a scientifically controlled process of long-term, in-depth study. Read Chapter 12, "Alternatives to MHT," for a full discussion of this issue, and be aware that you can't just stroll down the aisle of your local health food store and choose a safe, effective, natural cure for any of your hormonal symptoms based on the claims of the label.

The Search for Herbal Treatments

Doctors and scientists around the world continue to evaluate the effectiveness of some of the most popular alternative treatments for the symptoms of menopause because many women use them. While a great deal remains to be learned about the safety, effectiveness, and long-term value of these treatment options, some of the alternative treatments most commonly used for the relief of hot flashes include:

- **Soy products.** Soy products, including whole soy foods, soy protein capsules, and isoflavone extracts, offer some relief from mild hot flashes, according to the results of some studies. Soy proteins are available in soy milk, tofu, tempeh, and roasted soy nuts. Because researchers haven't determined how phytoestrogens in soy interact with cancerous cells, however, these products aren't recommended for women seeking nonhormonal relief from menopause symptoms due to a history of cancer. Studies typically show that while women do experience lessening of hot flashes when they increase soy intake, it is not significantly more than the relief they experience when taking placebo.

- **Vitamin E.** Some women have reported that taking vitamin E offered them relief from hot flashes. In studies where participants took a regulated daily dose of 800 international units of vitamin E, the women did experience some minor relief (on the order of one less hot flash per day), and the vitamin caused no negative side effects. Right now, no study supports the idea that you can achieve significant relief from hot flashes by taking vitamin E, but studies continue in this area.

Is Black Cohosh the Answer?

Black cohosh is a plant in the buttercup family whose root is used in the treatment of menopausal symptoms. It is popular in Europe as a treatment for premenstrual syndrome and a number of menopausal symptoms. Though some products containing extracts of black cohosh carry labels that claim they can reduce hot flashes by as much as 25 percent, many medical experts feel that data to verify the herb's effectiveness is lacking. Studies have shown mixed results, but a rigorous double-blind study done in 2006 reported that black cohosh had no more effect on hot flashes than placebo, even when combined with other herbal therapies. Although many women report some improvement with the use of this herb, studies still do not support its use for hot flashes.

 Fact

Research has not yet determined whether black cohosh is safe for women with breast cancer and other estrogen-sensitive cancers. If you suspect you may be pregnant, avoid taking black cohosh; it may cause miscarriage or premature birth.

When considering whether to try this herbal treatment, remember that it does have a number of negative side effects, including nausea and dizziness. When using black cohosh for the treatment of perimenopause or menopause symptoms, you should limit the total treatment time to no more than six months.

Mind-Body Exercises

Many women have found that they can limit the number and severity of hot flashes using mind-body practices such as yoga, meditation, visualization, and deep breathing. It is worth noting that in many menopause studies placebo works as well as many of the remedies being studied. This is a strong indicator that expectations—and your mind—have a profound effect on your body's responses. Stress, anxiety, and fatigue can contribute to the onset and severity of hot flashes; these techniques help calm the mind, relax your muscles and nerves, and keep you feeling rested and at ease. Even when hot flashes do occur, regular practice of these techniques can help you recover more quickly from their effects. And these relaxation techniques and mind-body exercises work to combat a number of other menopausal symptoms, including mood swings, sleeplessness, muscle loss, joint aches, and reduced cognitive functions.

Take a Deep Breath

Use deep breathing to calm a raging hot flash; practice it regularly to help avoid the onset of hot flashes throughout the day and night. Deep, paced breathing is a strong tool for calming the body and the mind—and it's an incredibly easy technique to use. If you feel a hot flash coming on, begin taking deep, slow breaths through your nose. Breathe in to expand your lungs as far as you can, then hold the breath there for a few seconds before you slowly release it. Let your belly swell out and your chest expand as you breathe in, so your body is fully "inflating" with the breath. When you exhale, empty your lungs completely. Take at least three full, deep breaths and try to remain calm.

Make It a Daily Habit

A daily program of meditation and relaxation is a powerful tool for keeping your body calm, focused, and strong throughout the day. Its stress-relieving benefits can help ward off hot flashes and other stress-related symptoms of menopause. A ten-minute relaxation session fits easily into your morning and evening schedule, and it's simple to do. Sit or lie down in a quiet place with your eyes closed. Consciously relax every muscle in your body, beginning with your feet and continuing the relaxation up toward your head. Concentrate on a single word or object that has personal meaning for you; if other ideas, worries, or mental chatter enter your mind, dismiss them and return to the thought of your focus word. After ten minutes, open your eyes, remain seated, and take three deep breaths before continuing with your day.

Essential

Use visualization techniques to help cool a hot flash. When you feel a hot flash begin to develop, close your eyes and envision being in a cool, breezy location. Think of the warmth as a liquid, and imagine that you can channel it to flow from your body. Envision the heat draining out through your hands and feet; then imagine that a cool layer of snow is falling on your head, shoulders, and arms.

Yoga: Not Just for Youngsters!

Yoga is an excellent practice for increasing flexibility, building muscle strength and endurance, and eliminating the negative effects of stress on your body. Practicing yoga stretches for twenty to thirty minutes three times a week can help reduce the negative effects of stress on your body, as it stretches your muscles, improves your balance, and encourages deep, full breathing. Regular yoga practice can also help reduce insomnia, so you fall asleep faster and stay asleep longer.

As you find your way through menopause, use your symptoms—including hot flashes—to increase your self-awareness. Talk to your health care provider, and try a combination of medicinal and mind-body suggestions until you find what best suits your symptoms and lifestyle. At the very least, you can reframe your hot flashes as "power surges" and keep a sense of humor about this temporary, if bothersome, phase.

CHAPTER 6

The New You—
Managing Physical
Changes

NOW THAT YOU CAN recognize the symptoms of menopause, what can be done? Many of the physical signs can be managed to improve your quality of life and make the transition more comfortable. This chapter will take a look at the physical symptoms described earlier and will offer options for making the most of your "new" self.

Irregular Periods

Since the very earliest sign of perimenopause is often a change in the regularity of your menstrual cycle, it's a good place to start on the list of physical menopausal changes. You may be one of those women who notice a change not only in the timing of your period, but also in the amount of flow. Sometimes heavier periods become so over several months or years, until one day you realize that your life revolves around having pads and tampons in every purse and coat pocket, and you begin to plan your vacations and activities around that time of the month. That is, if you can predict that time of the month.

What's Going On?

What causes cycle irregularity during perimenopause? Once again, the culprit behind the majority of irregular periods is hormonal fluctuations. In fact, hormone fluctuations can cause a variety of irregularities in your periods. As you enter perimenopause, you probably ovulate less frequently. Because all hormone releases are triggered by others, an unusual fluctuation in one hormone can set off a series of unusual fluctuations in others, as your body tries to spur on or hold back the hormone in flux. For that reason, you might have a six-week cycle, followed by a four-week cycle, followed by a six-week cycle with unusually light flow, and so on. (A cycle is the length of time from the first day of one menstrual period to the first day of the next.) Your body is going through a series of starts and stalls as it attempts to adjust to fluctuating levels of hormones in your bloodstream.

Because you ovulate less frequently during this time, your body's estrogen levels often are unchecked by progesterone. As a result, your uterine lining can develop abnormal cell changes that lead to unusually heavy bleeding or midcycle spotting.

Hyperplasia

A common cause of abnormal bleeding is a precancerous condition of the lining of the uterus called endometrial hyperplasia. This excessive growth of the uterine lining can result from having unbalanced estrogen. If diagnosed when still in its early stages, it can be treated medically. Untreated endometrial hyperplasia can develop into endometrial cancer. It's a good idea to report any changes in bleeding patterns to your health care provider.

Heavy Bleeding

As if unpredictable periods weren't enough, some women find that their periods become very heavy during perimenopause. This may be rather benign, and just a bit more bleeding than you have been always had; or it can mean significant blood loss, or be a sign of something serious. You may want to start counting the pads or tampons you use in a day and keep a note of it on your calendar, in case you need that information to discuss heavy bleeding with your health care provider.

Uterine Fibroids

As you've learned, unusual bleeding can have a number of causes, but two relatively common benign causes are fibroids and polyps. Uterine fibroids are benign growths of muscle tissue that develop within the wall of the uterus, on the uterine lining, or on the outside of the uterus. Also called leiomyomas, fibroids are extremely common and by age fifty as many as 80 percent of women have them. Fibroids within the uterine lining can cause abnormal bleeding because of the way they distort the lining and prevent it from shedding normally. Fibroids vary tremendously in size, from undetectable to the size of a grapefruit, or larger. Their size alone can cause problems, such as pelvic pressure, bloating, urinary frequency, or pain during intercourse. If you have unusually heavy or midcycle bleeding, your doctor probably will check for the presence of fibroids.

If your symptoms are found to be from fibroids, rather than from hormone fluctuations or other causes, your health care provider will probably recommend treating you. Treatment options for fibroids also vary, depending on the size of the tumors; whether you want to retain your fertility (not usually an issue during perimenopause, but it might be); and what resources are available in your area. Among the accepted treatments for uterine fibroids are the following:

- **"Wait and Watch."** Because these are benign growths, some health providers prefer to wait and monitor fibroids. This is acceptable if symptoms are not seriously affecting your life and health. Since fibroids usually shrink after menopause, this may be a good choice for women in perimenopause who are not having serious symptoms.

- **Embolization.** Fibroid tumors are dependent on the blood supply that develops around them, and in this procedure a specially trained radiologist injects a plastic or gelatin substance into the blood vessel through a small incision in the leg. A tube is inserted into the uterine artery, where particles are deposited on both sides of the artery, stopping the blood supply to the fibroid. It is relatively safe and can be done on an outpatient basis. Embolization is not usually recommended for women who want to remain fertile, since a pregnancy requires excellent blood supply to the uterus.

- **Medications.** There are several medication approaches to treating fibroids. You may be advised to take iron to treat anemia if you have been bleeding heavily. Or your doctor may prescribe non-steroidal anti-inflammatory medications (NSAIDs, such as ibuprofen, naproxen, etc.) for pain and inflammation and to decrease prostaglandin activity—this can decrease total menstrual blood loss by up to 50 percent. Oral contraceptives are used to decrease the bleeding, but they do not reduce the size of the fibroids. Because fibroids respond to a reduction of female hormones, sometimes androgens ("male" hormones) or a class of medications called gonadotropin-releasing hormone agonists may be used to reduce the action of estrogen and progesterone, thereby shrinking the tumors.

- **Myomectomy.** This is the surgical removal of the tumor itself, and is one choice for women who want to keep their uterus and are having significant symptoms of pain or bleeding. This treatment may be done by abdominal surgery or by laparoscope, and carries all the usual risks of those types of surgery.
- **Myolysis.** This treatment means using an electric current or liquid nitrogen to destroy the fibroid tissue. Done through a laparoscope, it seems to present fewer risks than abdominal surgery, but its safety and effectiveness are still being studied. It is not recommended for very large fibroids or for women who want to eventually become pregnant, since scarring and adhesions often follow the procedure.

 Alert

There is often cramping with fibroid embolization, and the pain may become severe as the fibroid tissue "dies" after the blood supply is cut off. This process of tissue death also increases the chance of infection. Although serious infection is rare, it can lead to hysterectomy. Be sure to explore the risks of this procedure before you decide to pursue it.

- **Focused Ultrasound Surgery (FUS).** FUS is the use of ultrasound to destroy fibroid tissue, and is done using a special magnetic resonance imaging (MRI) machine to locate and target the tumor. It is not yet well studied, but has promise as a less invasive form of surgery and is already being used for other procedures.
- **Hysterectomy.** Surgical removal of the uterus is the only certain way to eliminate fibroids and the symptoms they cause. It

is major surgery, however, and has its own set of risks and benefits, which must be considered before accepting it as the treatment of choice.

If you are diagnosed with fibroids and they are causing problems, discuss the options with your health care provider. He or she can help you weigh the seriousness of your symptoms with the risks and benefits of treatments.

 ## Fact

Uterine fibroids can cause bleeding serious enough to make you anemic. If you find during your period that you are changing a maxi-pad or super tampon more than eight times in eight hours, or if you have clots that last over eight hours, make an appointment with your health care provider to be evaluated for these benign but troublesome tumors.

Polyps

Uterine polyps are smaller benign growths on the lining of the uterus. Science and medicine have yet to explain why polyps develop in some women, and not in others. Polyps bleed, just like fibroids, but because they are typically small, they're unlikely to cause the amount of blood loss associated with fibroids. When a health care provider diagnoses polyps (usually through an ultrasound test or a biopsy sample), he or she can remove them through a simple outpatient procedure in which the doctor snips the polyps from the uterine lining. This procedure usually involves a hysteroscopy—a sophisticated dilation and curettage (D and C) procedure where a small (one-eighth-inch) camera lens and instrument port are inserted into the cervix to locate the polyps and remove all of them at that time. Although pain is usually minimal, you may receive mild sedation or anesthesia during the procedure, and some pain medication afterward.

Heart Palpitations

Heart palpitations are very common during perimenopause and are usually a bit startling the first couple of times they occur. Your heart may feel like it is racing, slowing, irregular, or just "thrashing around in there." It may accompany or precede a hot flash, and is probably responding to the same hormone fluctuations that make the rest of your vascular system a little unstable during this time. Because cardiac problems sometimes start in midlife, you will want to check with your health care provider if you have palpitations frequently or if they are painful or dramatic.

It's Not Love, It's the Coffee

Remember when a rapidly beating heart meant you were excited to see a new love? Menopausal palpitations can feel like that, but the most likely cause is either anxiety or stimulants. It's hard to say whether women feel anxious because their hearts are beating fast, or their hearts beat fast because they are anxious. If you find yourself feeling anxious or having panic episodes, talk to your health care provider or mental health counselor. There are relaxation exercises, biofeedback techniques, and medications that can help you through anxious moments or events.

And if you are a habitual stimulant user you may notice that heart palpitations may occur when you use alcohol, caffeine, diet pills, or decongestants. Even if you are used to these substances, they may set off an episode of palpitating because you're more sensitive to small changes, just as spicy food can trigger a hot flash.

Other medical conditions may have palpitations as a symptom, which is why it's a good idea to check out any changes in your heartbeat. If you are anemic, dehydrated, or have high blood sugar or an overactive thyroid, you may notice heart palpitations. Any of these conditions should be evaluated to be sure they are not serious health problems.

Is It a Heart Attack?

That, of course, is the fear when your heart starts acting erratically. Although cardiac disease is rarely the cause of heart palpitations in perimenopause, it is possible that you are experiencing cardiac symptoms. Heart attack symptoms are different for women than for men, and it is important not to dismiss ongoing heart irregularities without having them evaluated.

Like other transient symptoms of the perimenopause, palpitations usually go away on their own after a few months. If you find that exercise or certain situations trigger them, learn to stop what you are doing and breathe in a slow, regular way until your heartbeat returns to normal. This, too, shall pass.

 Alert

Although heart palpitations are common during perimenopause and are almost always benign, they can also signal more serious problems. If you have dizziness, fainting, tightness in the neck or chest, abdominal pain, or nausea with the palpitations, or if your heart rate is over 120 beats a minute, go to the emergency room or urgent care to be checked.

Involuntary Urine Release

Many women are subject to urinary tract infections (UTIs) on and off throughout their adult lives. But this problem can worsen during perimenopause. Estrogen contributes to the growth and nourishment of all cells and tissues. Because your body produces lower levels of estrogen during the years leading to menopause, the tissues lining the urinary tract can grow thin and more prone to bacterial infection and inflammation. That same lack of estrogen-induced nourishment can weaken the muscles that surround your bladder and urethra. As a result, you experience more UTIs and other urinary tract disorders, a weaker bladder, and less control over urine release.

The most common kinds of urinary tract disorders women experience during perimenopause are stress urinary incontinence, urge incontinence, and UTIs. These disorders can have similar symptoms, but their causes and treatments are very different.

Urinary Tract Infections

Urinary tract infections are caused by bacteria in the urinary tract. The symptoms of UTI include feeling as though you need to urinate all the time, even when your bladder is empty; a burning sensation during urination; and—infrequently—small amounts of blood in your urine. Urinary tract infections can seem to fade, then return again. It's important to remember that, as with any bacterial infections, a full-blown UTI won't go away without antibiotic treatment. If left unchecked, the bacteria that cause a simple bladder infection can spread to the kidneys, causing a much more serious infection called pyelonephritis.

 Fact

Many urinary tract disorders have similar symptoms, but require different treatments. If you suffer from burning or too frequent urination, involuntary urine release, or a constant full bladder feeling, see your doctor for an accurate diagnosis and treatment.

Urge Incontinence

Urge incontinence is the result of a bladder spasm that forces urine out, even when the bladder is not completely full. These involuntary muscle contractions cause the bladder to release urine in varying amounts. Even though the woman may not feel as though her bladder is full and she needs to urinate, the sight, sound, or even thought of water or urination can cause the sudden reflex need to urinate and an accompanying release of urine.

Stress Incontinence

Stress urinary incontinence is another cause of periodic involuntary urine release. Unlike urge incontinence that can result from the mere thought of emptying the bladder, stress incontinence usually has a specific triggering event, such as a sneeze or cough. Some women release small amounts of urine when they bend over, laugh, or exercise.

Stress urinary incontinence is caused by weakened sphincter muscles, which surround the urethra, and can occur in women of any age. Women who have given birth, regardless of the type of delivery, often experience this disorder many years before they approach menopause. But during menopause, weakening sphincter muscles can contribute to the onset of stress urinary incontinence, even in women who have never had a pregnancy. Obesity and chronic lung conditions that produce a lot of coughing, such as emphysema or cigarette smoking, can also cause or aggravate the condition. There are several approaches that seem to improve this condition, including:

- A specific strengthening exercise called the Kegel exercise
- Physical therapy with biofeedback and pessaries – small devices worn in the vagina to support the weakened urethral muscles
- Surgery
- Weight loss
- Quitting smoking

If you begin to notice stress urinary incontinence when you cough or laugh, talk to your health care provider about these treatments.

Essential

A number of therapies can help end many urinary tract disorders. Biofeedback, pelvic floor muscle exercises (known as Kegel exercises), and medication are just some treatment possibilities. Weight loss and bladder retraining can be successful tools in fighting incontinence, too. Talk with your doctor to learn more.

Weight Gain

Your body's metabolism changes as you move into middle age. As you age, your body burns calories much more slowly (some studies say by as much as 4 to 5 percent) as each decade passes. So, instead of burning off the calories that you eat, your body converts them into fat. You may feel as though you aren't eating any more, and may actually feel you are eating less, but your body's furnace just needs less fuel to perform the same functions.

Although you may think you are always on your feet and very active, many people slow down a bit as they move into middle age—running fewer errands, doing less physical work around the house, and so on. All of these factors contribute to unwanted weight gain during perimenopause and after menopause.

Beating the Odds

As if a slowing metabolism isn't enough of a challenge, there are other conditions of aging and menopause that may make weight gain more likely. First of all, you may be more sedentary as you get older. Your job may require being confined to a desk, or without kids to chase around you may find yourself sitting on the couch watching TV. This is not a pattern that helps you burn calories. And if you develop diabetes or have painful conditions like arthritis or joint pain, you will be even more reluctant to move around, thus slowing your metabolism even more.

Although it may seem discouraging to consider all the reasons that make it difficult to lose or maintain weight, it is also the perfect opportunity to take a hard look at how you want to live the next years of your life. This may be just the time that you finally decide to become more active and eat healthy foods, since you can't count on a young metabolism to take care of those extra calories. Diet and exercise are discussed later in this book, but weight gain is a physical symptom of menopause that you can address directly with enough support and information.

Is It All in My Genes?

Weight problems are so common in this country that you cannot pass a grocery checkout or newsstand without seeing numerous articles on weight loss (usually in the same magazines with recipes for cake!). Most people have an ambivalent relationship with food, using it to comfort, nourish, and reward themselves. At the same time, they aspire to be as willowy as the models they see on the covers of those same magazines. Your body weight is a combination of food habits, genetic makeup, and activity levels. It's true that you inherit many influences on your weight, such as tendencies to gain or not, how we process and burn calories, and likelihood of getting obesity-related diseases. You can't change your genetic makeup any more than you can change your eye color. But you do have control over what and how much you eat, how much you move, and your attitude toward fitness. Those "change-able" factors are the focus of later chapters, and they are your best bets for getting and keeping a healthy weight.

 ## Fact

If you find yourself gaining weight as you get older, you are not alone. About a third of adults in the United States are clinically "obese," and another third are "overweight." The percentage of obese adults has nearly doubled in the last twenty-five years. Use the supportive programs and information that have resulted from this epidemic to avoid becoming one of the statistics.

Other Physical Changes Associated with Menopause

After menopause, estrogen and progesterone levels plummet. Although other parts of your body continue to produce some hormones, they cannot compensate fully for the loss of ovarian hormone production. The specific role of these hormones is treated in Chapter 11. Some of the major postmenopausal side effects are increased bone loss and your skin tissues becoming thinner and less elastic. Your organs and joints respond to diminishing hormones as well as to the wear and tear of living.

Catching Up with Men—Not Always a Good Thing

After menopause, women are just as likely to develop heart disease as men are. Your cardiovascular system misses those hormones, too, with their beneficial impact on HDL cholesterol and their inhibiting effect on LDL cholesterol. With the loss of protective hormones, your arteries become more susceptible to plaque buildup, and begin to narrow and lose elasticity. As a result, estrogen loss can contribute to heart disease.

Boning Up on Osteoporosis

Another important side effect of plummeting hormones is a rapid advance of the bone loss that began in your forties. In the first five years that follow menopause, women can lose as much as one-fourth of their bone density—a potentially deadly development. Bone fractures that develop as a result of osteoporosis can have life-threatening consequences. This bone loss slows down for most women within a decade or so of menopause, but without supplements or MHT, it continues throughout a woman's life. There are ways to minimize this bone loss and the dangers it brings, and you will learn about them in Chapter 15.

More Postmenopausal Changes

During your fifties and early sixties—the decades immediately following menopause—your body undergoes some inevitable changes resulting from the natural aging process. Your body is unique, and so are your family medical history, your lifestyle, and your individual health program. In general, here are the types of changes many women experience in the years that follow menopause:

- Hearing loss can set in, due to the ear canal tissue's becoming thinner and drier. Many people have no hearing loss until they are in their sixties, but almost one-third of women over sixty-five report hearing problems. Keep this loss to a minimum by protecting your ears from loud noises. Wear earplugs when you mow the lawn and avoid sitting close to loud stereos and televisions. And get annual hearing checkups, so you know when your hearing loss reaches the you-need-a-hearing-aid stage.
- Joints lose cartilage with age and connective tissue becomes less flexible and resilient, making arthritis and other types of joint pain more common in aging women. Exercise and weight control are critical factors in maintaining healthy joints.

- Lungs become less elastic as we hit our mid-fifties, which can contribute to shallower breathing and, therefore, less oxygen in our bloodstream. Get plenty of aerobic exercise to keep your lungs pumping. If you're still smoking, quit now!
- The brain loses mass and shrinks slightly with each passing year. As a result, women can face impaired cognitive functions as early as age seventy. Keep your body and mind active— participate in a regular aerobic exercise program, work cross-word puzzles, learn to use the computer, visit with family and friends, read the newspaper, and travel. Life's pleasures are also your best weapon in keeping your mind alert and agile.
- Digestion slows down as you reach your sixties, and food moves at a slower pace through your intestines. As a result, many post-menopausal women report problems with constipation. Eat plenty of whole grains, fresh fruit, and vegetables, and drink plenty of water to combat this change in your digestive function and, you guessed it, exercise.

Living for the Rest of Your Life

These changes contribute to the challenges you face in maintaining your strength and health as you move through the postmenopausal years of your life. Though aging is inevitable, you have tremendous control over its effects. Menopause is great training for learning how to age because it demands that you pay attention to your body, make decisions, and take actions that can protect and nurture it throughout the many years ahead. Learning how to take control of your health and choices is worth the effort because menopause also can usher in a time of great freedom, personal exploration, and growth. How you manage the symptoms of perimenopause and the realities of aging that follow will determine your own postmenopausal experience. The remaining chapters of this book take a closer look at all the health issues that surround menopause, and offer simple, effective, ideas for managing your health and combating these issues—now and for the rest of your life.

CHAPTER 7

Managing Cognitive and Neurological Changes

NEXT TO HOT FLASHES, the menopause symptoms that bother women the most are the ones involving their brains. If you find your memory seems to be lapsing or you have some trouble concentrating, it can be unsettling or even alarming. Women ask themselves, "Am I going crazy? Do I have Alzheimer's? And where are those car keys anyway?" This chapter will cover neurological symptoms and some treatments that may offer you that much needed relief.

My Mind—Where Did It Go?

If you're nearing age fifty and you haven't yet begun to experience periodic memory lapses, consider yourself lucky. The busier and more stressful life becomes, the easier it is to misplace items, forget an associate's name, lose track of the point you were about to make, and remember the title of that movie. As one fifty-something friend once said, "It takes three middle-aged people to tell any one story." Multiple events challenge the memory at middle age and many of them still are not fully understood. Though many women wonder if they're showing the first signs of Alzheimer's, the vast majority of memory loss problems are natural—and sometimes transient—responses to the effects of age, menopausal hormone changes, stress, and a busy, changing life.

Memory Problems

Many women report an increase in forgetfulness and memory loss, as well as decreased mental clarity, during perimenopause. Because hormones tend to fluctuate dramatically during this period, estrogen deficiency used to be the culprit most often blamed for changes in memory functions. But studies such as the Seattle Midlife Women's Health Study, conducted by the University of Washington in 2000, dispute that notion. In that study, researchers found that neither the age nor the perimenopausal stage of the women studied were linked to any diminishment of the women's mental functions. In fact, the study found that younger women and women undergoing hormone therapy were more likely than midlife women to report problems with memory loss.

 Fact

Alzheimer's disease is more common in women than in men, and it strikes women at an earlier age. The symptoms, which include memory loss, diminished language and motor skills, and an inability to recognize people or objects, appear gradually and worsen with age. If you are increasingly dependent on others for your decisions, or are losing the ability to do everyday tasks, you can ask your health care provider to perform diagnostic tests to see if you have early Alzheimer's disease.

The Seattle study found that physical health, emotional factors, and stress accounted for almost half of the memory loss noted in participants. Depression and high levels of stress played a key role in short-term memory degradation. Among participants in the study, only 24 percent of memory loss was attributed to the physical effects of aging.

Most medical and scientific authorities agree that age results in subtle changes in anyone's ability to think clearly and quickly, but that doesn't link memory loss to menopause; causes for these mental lapses are tied more closely to the brain than the ovaries. First, the human brain shrinks after age fifty, due to a loss of water content. That shrinkage doesn't necessarily impair memory, of course, but a loss of volume in the frontal lobes can. Some neuroscientists say that the frontal lobes can shrink as much as 30 percent between the ages of fifty and ninety. Because the frontal lobes are so important to complex thinking, losses in that area of the brain can impair your ability to reason things out, maintain attention span, multitask, and use your best judgment.

Ⅼ Essential

Although you don't have to fear that your brain will shrink up like a walnut when you hit fifty, real physical changes can begin at this time, and you may begin to feel their impact on your short-term memory, attention span, and other thinking processes. Chapter 18 offers some simple techniques for keeping your mental edge as you move toward and through menopause.

And the brain's hippocampus can lose some of its capabilities with age, too. This part of the brain is responsible for creating, storing, and retrieving memory, and scientists now think it can lose a portion of those abilities with age. A slowing of mental processes accounts for many of the cognitive changes that you perceive with age. In other words, the information is all there and your brain can retrieve it—that retrieval process just takes longer than it used to. Metabolic changes and a diminished number of brain signal transmitters (called dendrites) on your brain cells (neurons) contribute to the slowdown.

Difficulty Concentrating

The inability to focus is also common in perimenopause, and may be due to normal aging of the brain or may be a temporary shift as your hormones change. There are several causes of decreased concentration, any or all of which may explain why you keep reading that paragraph over and over and can't seem to focus on the story you are reading.

Concentration, like memory, is a cognitive task that relies on brain chemicals and brain structures that are sensitive to hormonal changes. If you have a history of premenstrual syndrome (PMS) and found that you could not concentrate as well just before your period, you may be more prone to this symptom in menopause. As estrogen decreases, some women have fewer of the neurotransmitters such as serotonin to carry messages in the brain. And normal aging of the brain means that in middle age people become less able to turn off the "daydreaming" area of the brain, making it easier to be distracted and harder to pay attention.

As frustrating as it is to lose concentration, the news is not all bad. As your body adjusts to new levels of hormones, some of your ability to concentrate will return. And research is discovering that the human brain is much more adaptable than previously thought. When we lose abilities in one section of the brain, we seem to be able to rebuild those abilities using another part of the brain. The secret seems to lie, in part, with keeping your body and attitude healthy so that you have the right building materials to make those changes. More on this in Chapter 18.

 Fact

The level of stress hormones in your body can seriously alter your memory and concentration. Other factors such as loss of sleep, alcohol use, and vitamin B12 deficiency—all common during this life stage—are more common reasons for cognitive trouble than low estrogen.

Insomnia and Its Role in Menopause

Insomnia is a typical symptom of perimenopause, and it plays an active cause-and-effect role in other perimenopausal conditions. Night sweats and panic attacks, for example, can contribute to insomnia. Long-term insomnia can contribute to heightened anxiety and feelings of fatigue, moodiness, and irritability. When women don't get enough rest, they can have difficulty with concentration, focus, and memory, and their overall physical and mental health can suffer.

Insomnia—a condition characterized by an inadequate amount or poor quality of sleep occurring three or more nights a week—isn't a concern just of menopausal women. As a nation, the United States appears to have entered a time of greater sleeplessness than ever before. The National Sleep Foundation (NSF) (an independent, nonprofit organization) released the results of its own national sleep survey in 2003, revealing that 71 percent of American adults between the ages of 55 and 74 report some sort of sleep problem, and most say they were able to get more sleep in the past (as little as five years earlier) than at the time of the survey.

Menopausal women are at particular risk for insomnia. In a 2006 Harris poll, women suffering from insomnia reported that this was the symptom of menopause that bothered them the most, with 72 percent of participants experiencing it frequently (at least once per week), and 59 percent losing on average three or more hours of sleep each night. The vast majority of these women, 88 percent, said they have more fatigue during the day, 62 percent said they are more irritable, and 44 percent said they cannot do their job as well.

Hormonal Imbalances and Sleeplessness

Remember when you were a teenager and could—if allowed—sleep past noon? For most women approaching menopause, that capacity for endless sleep is only a distant memory. Throughout her adult life, a woman's hormonal balance affects her ability to sleep. Many women experience sleep disturbances during menstruation, pregnancy, and in perimenopause and menopause.

Women who experience PMS often report sleeping difficulties during that same late phase of the menstrual cycle (days 22 through 28). The physical symptoms of PMS include bloating, headache, moodiness, and cramping—all of which can contribute to sleeplessness. But women with PMS report a range of sleep problems in addition to insomnia, including hypersomnia (sleeping too much) and daytime sleepiness. As women who have a history of PMS approach menopause, those symptoms can become even more severe.

Essential

Women who are healthy sleepers spend 15 to 20 percent of their sleeping hours in deep sleep. Some research has suggested that women who have PMS may spend only 5 percent of their sleeping hours in deep sleep all month long.

Many sleep problems in perimenopause are caused by other symptoms of diminishing hormones, including hot flashes and night sweats. Though these problems may not diminish the length of a woman's sleep cycle, they can disrupt sleep frequently enough to cause fatigue and sleepiness throughout the following day. In the NSF poll, women reported that hot flashes contributed to their sleep disturbances at least five days a month.

Many doctors recommend hormone therapy or alternative treatments to combat many of the symptoms of perimenopause and menopause, including sleeplessness.

 Alert

Six in ten adults in the United States say they experience frequent sleep problems. In the National Sleep Survey of 2001, a high percentage of those with certain health problems common to perimenopause experienced sleep problems, including depression (83 percent), nighttime heartburn (82 percent), and hypertension (79 percent).

Understanding and Treating Sleep Problems

Hormonal imbalances aren't the only cause of sleep disruption for women in perimenopause and menopause. Depression and anxiety are common contributors to sleeplessness. Remember, these problems feed each other. The less rested you are, the more powerful your negative feelings become, and the less able you are to see your way through them. Stress—an enemy of women at any age—can also severely inhibit your ability to enjoy deep, restful sleep. A late-night trip to the bathroom, for example, may be followed by hours of sleeplessness brought on by stress-induced worry. If you awaken due to pain, or have a tendency to "snap" awake at 4 a.m. for no good reason, and lie in bed worrying about vague concerns or relatively inconsequential issues until the alarm goes off at 7 A.M., stress is playing a role in your sleep disturbance. All of these triggers can combine to create a powerful enemy of your good health as you approach and pass through menopause.

Chapter 8 offers you some valuable techniques for recognizing and combating stress and emotional states that can contribute to (and feed on) sleeplessness. Acknowledging that sleep disturbance is part of this overall pattern is an important first step in any treatment. The next step is to talk with health professional about these problems and their solution.

Your sleep problems may have nothing to do with stress, anxiety, or tension, but could have physical sources. One in four women over fifty, for example, suffers from sleep apnea, a sleep disorder in which the sleeper stops breathing for frequent, short periods throughout the night. Snoring and daytime sleepiness are clues that you might be suffering from sleep apnea. Snoring can increase with weight gain—particularly when you gain weight around your neck. If you have a problem with daytime sleepiness and your partner complains that your snoring is becoming louder, see your doctor. Sleep apnea is associated with other medical problems, including high blood pressure and cardiovascular disease, so it isn't something to blow off (so to speak).

More women than men suffer pain-related sleep problems. Pain from arthritis, migraine headaches, tension, chronic fatigue syndrome, and fibromyalgia have been linked to sleep disruption in women. Pain can make falling asleep and staying asleep more difficult, but many people fail to report (or recognize) sleeplessness as a problem. If pain is interrupting your sleep, ask your health care professional about pain management options.

 Fact

Rapid Eye Movement (REM) sleep is the most active sleep state—the one in which dreams occur. Scientists divide non-REM sleep (about 80 percent of total sleep) into four stages. In each stage, brain waves grow larger and slower. After the fourth stage, the deepest period of sleep, the brain waves reverse the pattern; sleep progresses toward its lightest stage, REM sleep. Typically, the cycle takes about ninety minutes.

Travel can wreak havoc with sleep quality and quantity, too. Many menopausal and perimenopausal women are in professional positions that require them to travel frequently. Hopping from time zone to time zone, spending long hours in airports and on planes, and sleeping in one hotel after another can seriously damage the quality and quantity of anyone's sleep. If you're already dealing with fluctuating hormones and subsequent hot flashes, night sweats, and periodic anxiety attacks, this kind of disruption can make your sleep problems even more severe.

 Alert

> If you or your partner is a heavy snorer, or have other risk factors for sleep apnea, your symptoms could cause sleep problems for both of you. Sleep apnea is a serious condition and can contribute to overweight and heart disease. Your primary care physician can refer you to a sleep study medical center that can help diagnose the problem and recommend treatment.

IsYour Lifestyle Keeping You Awake?

Simple lifestyle choices may be at the root of many sleep disturbances. Although you may be following the same practices you've followed for years, as your body changes in perimenopause and menopause, you may have to become more protective of your body's natural ability to sleep. Here are some of the most common daily habits that can interfere with good, restful sleep:

- **Alcohol.** You may think a nightcap will help you sleep, but it probably won't. Drinking alcohol right before bedtime may help you fall asleep, but it's also likely to wake you up hours before you're ready to rise. Avoid alcohol for at least two to four hours before heading for bed.

- **Caffeine.** Caffeine can stimulate your brain and make it difficult for you to go to sleep and stay asleep. Limit the amount of caffeine you consume during the day, and confine that consumption to the morning or early afternoon hours. Or cut out the caffeine altogether.

- **Exercising at night.** Yes, exercise is essential for good health, but it's a powerful mind and body stimulant. Exercise regularly to help put your body on a natural schedule, but don't exercise in the two to three hours before bedtime.

- **Smoking.** Nicotine is a stimulant. As you already know, your good health requires that you quit altogether. If you continue to smoke, however, stop at least two to three hours before bedtime.

- **Your sleep environment.** If your partner snores; if your cat or dog walks all over you through the night; if your room is too hot, too cold, too noisy, or too bright, you won't sleep well. Keep the sleeping room temperature between 65 and 70 degrees. Use light-blocking window shades or wear a sleep mask. And finally, consider sleeping apart from disruptive sleep partners of any species (a difficult step, but perhaps essential).

Putting Sleep Disorders to Rest

You can't control your body's evolution, and you probably aren't willing to tell your boss, "No travel until after menopause," so what can you do? The most important way to promote and protect healthy sleep patterns is to pay attention to sleep problems when they arise and then take action to resolve them. If the lifestyle changes suggested in the preceding section don't alleviate your sleep problems, seek professional help. Although polls report that many people describe sleep problems as common experiences, many of those same people will say that they don't suffer from sleep disorders. You may think that missing an hour or two of sleep now and then isn't a problem, but if you aren't getting enough sleep—and that means at least eight hours a day for most adults—your physical and emotional health will suffer.

Prescription Medications

You and your medical provider may decide that your insomnia is serious enough to warrant trying medication. There are a number of choices, depending on your history and the severity of your insomnia. Some of the choices are:

- **Hypnotic-Sedatives.** These valium-like medications help with falling and staying asleep. Older types can be habit forming, while newer "non-benzodiazapine" hypnotics seem to be as effective without being habit forming. None of these are recommended for long-term use.
- **Sedating antidepressants.** These are usually the "tricyclic" antidepressants. While they do have some uncomfortable side effects, they are sometimes chosen because they also help with pain management, and may be a good choice for treating depression and insomnia at the same time.
- **Over-the-counter sedatives.** These are typically some form of antihistamine, and may be useful for occasional insomnia, but their "hangover" effects of sleepiness and motor impairment need to be evaluated for their impact on your ability to function well the day after using them.

So, if you have trouble falling asleep or are awakening frequently during the night, and none of the lifestyle changes you've made have helped, talk to a health care professional. You have a number of options for resolving sleep problems, including changing your diet or exercise schedule, medications, hormone therapy, relaxation techniques, biofeedback, and psychological counseling. Though sleep disturbances may be a short episode in your passage to menopause, you shouldn't allow them to get the upper hand—for any length of time. Protect your sleep so that you can protect your health.

Headaches

Headaches are a common perimenopausal symptom. Some women will experience migraine headaches for the first time during this period, or a worsening of a long-standing migraine condition. Others will notice an increase in tension headaches. Whether it is migraine or tension, a headache can seriously limit your productivity and well-being.

Migraine Headaches

Migraine headaches are vascular, and are caused by blood vessels in the head enlarging, and then nerves around the blood vessels releasing chemicals that cause inflammation and pain. This migraine event usually triggers the "sympathetic" nervous system, the so-called "fight or flight" response, and thereby may cause nausea, vomiting, and diarrhea.

Since migraine headaches are sensitive to hormone shifts, women tend to have more of them during times when hormones fluctuate, such as the premenstruum, pregnancy, and menopause. They can be little more than a nuisance, or they can be debilitating events that put you out of commission for days at a time.

 Fact

As many as 20 percent of migraine headaches are immediately preceded by an "aura" or sensory change. The aura may be a visual change such as flashing lights or a blind spot in the visual field, a "pins and needles" sensation on one side, or even a strange taste or sound. This aura is sometimes enough of a heads-up that medication can be started in time to diminish the headache.

Some women experience an advanced warning other than an aura that comes days or hours before the headache. It may take any of a number of forms, including:

- Irritability
- Sadness
- Euphoria
- Sleepiness
- Yawning
- Food cravings

People with this sort of migraine learn to heed the warning and seek treatment before the headache hits. Often there are triggers for migraine headaches, including foods (aged cheese, coffee, chocolate, pickled items, and others), changes in sleep patterns (too much or too little), stress, artificial sweeteners such as aspartame, fasting, odors, alcohol, food additives such as monosodium glutamate (MSG), bright and flashing lights, and others. Sometimes avoiding triggers is effective in reducing the headaches significantly.

There are many ways to treat migraine headaches, some of them requiring prescription and some available over the counter. Combining caffeine with common pain medications is effective for some. Others find that they need to try prescription medications such as triptans or ergot formulas. Talking to your health care provider is important to determine which medications are best for you, and which will not interact badly with other medications you may be taking.

Non-medication approaches for migraine headaches include relaxation techniques and biofeedback. Ice can be effective in aborting headaches, and getting sufficient sleep is also important in preventing migraine attacks.

Essential

If you notice an increase in migraine headaches with menopause, see your health care provider. He or she can help you choose prevention and treatment options, and can sort out whether this change is related to a more serious medical condition, such as stroke or neurological disease.

Non-Migraine Headaches

A non-migraine headache is usually called a "tension headache." As with migraines, these are more common in women than men, and often begin in middle adulthood. Tension headaches, as the name implies, seem to result in the muscular tension in the neck and shoulders. As life, work and family become increasingly stressful, women notice more severe and more frequent tension headaches. Tension headaches may be associated with anxiety or depression, and are often treated successfully.

Treatment of tension headaches may be with common pain medications such as ibuprofen or acetaminophen, or with relaxation techniques and biofeedback, or some combination of the two. The most effective approach also is one that reduces the stress that causes the headache to begin with (more about stress management in Chapter 8). Some women find that chiropractic care, acupuncture, and/or massage can significantly reduce the number or severity of their tension headaches.

 Alert

A headache that comes on suddenly after the age of fifty can be a sign of serious illness. If you are a regular headache sufferer who notices a change in your headache pattern; if you have never had headaches and suddenly begin to have them; if your headache lasts for more than a day; or if your headache is not relieved with simple pain relievers, see your medical provider right away.

Dizziness

Although it is not known exactly why, many women find that they have episodes of dizziness during the perimenopause. The dizziness can range from just a slight sensation of "room spinning" to debilitating nausea or vertigo that affects your ability to walk.

There are several causes that might account for dizziness at this time of life. In most cases, it is likely to be one of the following:

- **Hyperventilation.** Stress or anxiety can trigger shallow breathing, which can cause your arteries to constrict. This loss of blood to your brain and extremities can make you light-headed and can cause your hands and feet feel to be numb. Taking long, slow, deep breaths may reduce the dizziness.

Fact

> Dizziness can be a side effect of many medications, including anti-depressants, blood pressure medicines, heartburn medications, sedatives, antihistamines, and decongestants. If you are taking any of these medications, check with your pharmacist or health care provider to see if dizziness is a side effect.

- **Low blood sugar levels.** If you are dieting rigorously, or just busy and not paying attention to mealtimes, you may have a drop in blood sugar that makes you feel light-headed. If this is common for you, schedule frequent snacks containing some protein with complex carbohydrates—such as cheese and whole-wheat crackers.
- **Hypotension.** If you notice dizziness when you stand up quickly, it's possible that you are having a drop in blood pressure when you stand. Change positions slowly, and increase your water intake, since being dehydrated can make your blood pressure even lower.

More Serious Possibilities

Although dizziness is common in the perimenopause, it can also be caused by serious conditions that need to be evaluated. Stroke, Parkinson's disease, cancerous tumors, vestibular disorders, and multiple sclerosis are all conditions that may have dizziness as a symptom. If you have dizziness that came on suddenly, impacts your ability to perform day-to-day activities, has other neurological symptoms along with it, or persists for weeks, see your health care provider about possible causes.

Other Neurological Symptoms

Because hormones can have such wide-ranging effects on the brain and nervous system, women report many symptoms that are not always found on the "typical signs of menopause" lists. But if they are, in fact, due to the changing levels of estrogen, these troublesome symptoms will be temporary and disappear as your body adjusts to new hormone levels.

Tinnitus

Tinnitus is defined as "ringing in the ears," but it has also been described as whooshing, roaring, chirping, pulsing, and screeching. It can be any persistent noise that a person hears, but that is not generated outside the body. While women sometimes begin to notice it with the onset of perimenopause, it has also been associated with other hormone shifts such as puberty and pregnancy. It is not clear how much of this symptom is related to the change in hormone levels, and how much is the result of getting older. By the age of sixty-five, a third of women will report that they have tinnitus at least now and then.

 Alert

> Be aware that although often benign, tinnitus can also signal a serious medical condition such as heart disease or thyroid problem. It can also be a side effect of medications including hormone therapy, antidepressants, and pain medications. Be sure to report it to your health care practitioner when discussing your symptoms.

One cause may be otosclerosis, which is a stiffening or hardening of the bones in the ear and can lead to loss of hearing. Tinnitus has also been reported as a side effect of menopausal hormone therapy, and has been related to fluid retention. There is no well-defined treatment for tinnitus, but here are some things you can do to help reduce it:

- Avoid loud sounds or excessively noisy environments.
- Decrease your intake of sodium/salt.
- Avoid stimulants such as caffeine and nicotine.
- Have your blood pressure checked to be sure it is within normal range.
- Get adequate exercise to increase blood flow to all of your body.

- Get enough sleep.
- Use "white noise" machines to make tinnitus less bothersome when trying to fall asleep.
- Practice relaxation or biofeedback exercises to reduce stress.
- Avoid aspirin or other pain medications in the non-steroidal anti-inflammatory (NSAID) family such as ibuprofen and naproxen.

Tingling/Burning and Other Paresthesias

A paresthesia is a skin sensation without an apparent physical cause. These sensations are reported by women in perimenopause, and can be unsettling. They take many forms, and may be described as numbness, pricking, burning, tingling, creepy crawly, pins and needles, or electric shocks; some women describe feeling "cobwebby" or feeling that they have "ants under the skin." It is thought that they are the result of vasomotor instability, the same mechanism that brings you hot flashes. In fact, some women get a paresthesia just before a hot flash, as a sort of warning. Paresthesia may also be caused by the hyperventilation that some women experience with panic or anxiety attacks. Whatever the cause, they are usually transitory, and seem to improve after actual menopause occurs.

Some women experience facial paresthesias that signal a oncoming migraine headache. Most paresthesias are more emotionally disturbing than physically dangerous. But since multiple sclerosis and some neurological conditions have this as a symptom, you should report it to your medical provider.

You're Not Crazy!

This chapter has described many neurological and cognitive symptoms that occur during menopause. As with all menopausal symptoms, these are interrelated with your health and lifestyle, and must be considered as part of the larger picture of perimenopause. Your emotional health, physical health, and life situation all influence how your symptoms will express themselves. Realize that these symptoms change as you go through the perimenopause and that you are not "going crazy." As with adolescence, your shift in hormones may cause changes that, although hard to keep up with, are perfectly normal.

Overcoming Mood Swings, Anxiety, and Depression

MANY WOMEN EXPERIENCE depression, anxiety, and/or mood swings during perimenopause. Mood disorders can be triggered by many things, and if you suffer from them—at any time during your life—it's important to understand where these problems come from as well as the best ways to treat them. Through medical treatment, stress management, and smart lifestyle choices, you can learn ways to regain control of your emotional stability.

Menopause and Emotions

Fluctuating hormones can cause emotional shifting. As anyone who has experienced premenstrual swings can understand, the effect of variable hormones on a woman's emotional stability can be unpredictable and unnerving. It's not just that your mood and behavior shift, but it's how they shift and how fast they shift that can leave you wondering what hit you.

"I'm Feeling Hormonal"

Women are used to the jokes and comments that people make about "that time of the month." Medical professionals are still studying and exploring the many ways hormones affect neurological processes, and in turn how women feel emotionally. It is usually the steroid hormones like estrogen, progesterone, and testosterone that get the attention around reproductive changes like menarche, puberty, and menopause. But there are many other hormones that change during these times and interact with brain functions, and these changes can cause strong emotional and behavior reactions.

Don't Kill the Messengers

Hormones are essentially chemical messengers designed to enter the bloodstream and serve some specific purpose. Since they have many different purposes such as reproduction, growth, or regulating the metabolism, it is not surprising that one of the areas they act on is the brain and its functions. So when one "family" of hormones changes, as when estrogen begins to decrease, it has a larger effect as other chemical messengers shift to keep things in balance. In the process of all this shifting around, some messages can get a little scrambled. If those scrambled messages alter your neurological processes, you may experience unfamiliar or unwanted emotional states.

Most of these changes are temporary if they are adjustments to your perimenopausal metabolism. But temporary or not, they can be upsetting and stressful if they show up as episodes of sadness, or rage, or even irritability. Some women experience many emotional variations during this phase, and some glide through without noticing much difference at all.

Mood Swings

Researchers believe that the fluctuating levels of estrogen and progesterone many women experience during this time contribute to mood swings and other emotional symptoms, though there are no clear conclusions about how this happens. Doctors know, however, that estrogen is directly related to our body's production of serotonin—an important chemical that works in the brain to regulate moods. As estrogen levels shift, so does the brain's supply of serotonin—and therefore, moods can shift, as well.

But body chemistry isn't the only thing that can trigger midlife mood decay. Women who are dealing with changing roles at home or at work or changing levels of energy, or who feel less fit or less healthy, may suffer from emotional upheavals and imbalances. Coming to grips with your emotional upsets by recognizing symptoms and tracking them to their source can be a first step toward solving the problem.

Which Comes First?

Just as mood swings in perimenopause can have both physical and emotional consequences, the causes of those mood swings can be both physical and emotional. First, consider that many of the symptoms of perimenopause can cause emotional distress. Hot flashes can lead to sleeplessness, fatigue, irritability, and anxiety. Those factors alone can make you feel angry, isolated, and under siege—and may contribute to occasional moodiness and transient depression. It is sometimes hard to sort out whether your moods swing because of other symptoms, or those symptoms come from your unpredictable reactions.

 Fact

> Mood swings are characterized by strong and sometimes rapidly changing emotional events. Women approaching menopause may report anxiety and panic attacks, bouts of sadness, or unexplained surges of elation. These emotional swings tend to be erratic and transient, not long-lived facts of life for perimenopausal women.

Tracking Your Mood Swings

Mood shifts are relatively mild changes in mood that can quickly take a woman from feelings of joy to anger, fatigue, or despair. The triggers for these responses can be unpredictable—and sometimes seemingly inconsequential. Perimenopausal women who report mood swings cite a wide range of stimuli for these events. If you're swinging, you can be moved to tears by a song on the radio or the color of the light as evening falls over your backyard. You can become incredibly angry when a coworker asks for clarification of a point you made in a memo, when children or a partner fail to take care of their household responsibilities, or when you forget to stop and pick up the dry cleaning on your way home. Mood swings can sometimes be no more than a typical response, but more intensely felt.

You may be reacting to some source of irritation, unhappiness, discomfort, fear, love, joy, or longing. As estrogen levels rise and fall, serotonin levels can rise and fall, too, taking your mood right along with them. Mood swings can also be a response to a medical condition or chemical imbalance in your body—one, that might be treatable through counseling, medication, or other therapy. Your mood swings can teach you a lot about who you are, what issues and changes you're dealing with, and where you want to go during this transition in your life.

You can expect some mood swings in your life, but many women in perimenopause develop mood swings that interfere with their daily living. Frequent or severe mood swings can create problems with family, coworkers, and friends. They can cause missed workdays, discourage participation in social functions or enjoyable activities, or create feelings of alienation, exhaustion, fear, and a lack of control. If mood swings are severe or frequent enough to get in the way of your full—and fulfilling—life, take action to bring them under control.

Essential

To get a handle on your mood swings, try tracking them for a month. Use a 1–5 scale, where 1 = happy and on track, and 5 = extremely negative, angry or sad. Record your mood at given times during the day or any times you notice changes. After recording for a month, look over your "mood map" and see if there are any patterns. Then talk to your health care provider about what might help.

Looking Stress in the Eye

Stress is a fact of life for everyone, and women approaching the age of menopause certainly aren't immune to its effects. In fact, women in perimenopause may be more susceptible to the health-damaging side effects of stress than they had been previously.

Women in midlife can be faced with career and financial issues, body-image changes, emerging health problems, divorce, widowhood, struggles with teenage children, and increasing responsibilities for aging parents. The added stress of adjusting to hormonal fluctuations, hot flashes, weight gain, or other potential side effects of perimenopause can make the burden of stress even harder to bear.

Fact

> Your stress may be connected to a medical condition or to the medication or treatment program you're using to combat one. Your doctor or health care provider may be able to adjust your medication or offer additional treatment options that can help you reduce and manage any health-related stressors you're encountering.

Some of the most common symptoms of stress include headaches, sleeplessness, indigestion, forgetfulness, an inability to concentrate, and ongoing feelings of anger and unhappiness. Stress can leave you feeling drained of all good feeling, and it can lead to overeating, drinking too much alcohol, or intensifying other unhealthy stress habits such as cigarette smoking. If you experience any of these symptoms of stress, you may have a real, health-threatening problem and can take action to determine its sources and potential solutions. Unless you find ways to eliminate or manage stress, you won't be successful in combating the mood-related problems you may experience during perimenopause.

Managing Stress

You can't avoid all sources of stress, but you may be able to find workarounds for many of them. If a hectic work and family schedule is depleting your energy and stressing you out, what can you trim from your list of daily activities? Can you ask a partner for help in managing household tasks or running errands? Can you afford to hire a service to do laundry, pick up and deliver dry cleaning, or take over major cleaning jobs around the house? If you have children, can you ask them to step up and take more responsibility for their own needs, or to help out more around the house? If aging parents are presenting increasing demands on your time, can you get any type of community support assistance, such as meal deliveries or the services of a visiting nurse?

Alert

Stress can trigger the biological changes that accompany depression, and it appears that hormonal shifts can trigger those changes, too. That's why women with a family or personal history of depression must be particularly careful to monitor and manage stress as they approach the age of menopause.

Gettinga Handle on Work Stressors

Evaluate your job and work habits to try to spot stress fixes there, as well. Can you ask your boss for flexible work times, so you can schedule your commute when traffic is less hectic, or even arrange to work at home one day a week? Can you find someone to carpool with? If you commute by train, can you do some of your work on a laptop computer and save time at the office? If you have problems with a coworker, can you schedule a meeting to try to resolve the issues, or at least to lessen the tension? Can a personal organizer, meeting scheduler program, or other software help you save time and cut down on unnecessary panic and last-minute emergencies?

Once you've pinpointed and reduced the stressors that you can, find ways to cope with the stress you can't avoid. Exercise regularly, spend time engaged in leisure activities you enjoy, eat a healthy diet, and go easy on your mind and body—don't expect to perform every task perfectly and on time.

The first key to addressing stress is to admit that stress is a real health risk—one you simply cannot overlook. Stress will wear you out, age your body and mind, drain your spirit, and cause lasting health problems. Though you may feel that you're stuck with the stressful situations you currently endure, you do have options available to you. Talk to your doctor, a therapist, a counselor, a friend, a minister, or a trusted family member, and ask for help in finding ways to manage stress.

Anxiety

Anxiety is a natural, healthy response to certain realities of life—beginning a new job, meeting upcoming deadlines, passing examinations, and so on. But anxiety that interferes with your ability to function throughout your day and then sleep soundly through the night is definitely unhealthy. Anxiety can be a side effect of a more serious mood-destabilizing condition—depression.

The Symptoms of Anxiety

Anxiety can be associated with depression, or it can be a side effect of sleeplessness, excess fatigue, or unmanageable levels of stress. Many people suffering from anxiety describe it as overwhelming feelings of fear, nervousness, or the conviction that something dreadful is about to happen—though they often can't pinpoint what that something may be. When these feelings begin to interfere with normal, everyday functioning, they may signal an anxiety disorder. Some other symptoms of anxiety include:

- An unshakable feeling of fear, dread, or worry that lasts for more than three days
- Chest pain, racing heart, or fast breathing
- Stomach pain, cramps, or diarrhea
- Hand wringing, pacing, or other repetitive nervous movement

Essential

Two important skills for decreasing stress are setting priorities and delegating. Take a look at responsibilities and decide which ones are truly essential. Women tend to think they have to do everything, without considering what is essential and what is optional. Once you have set priorities, delegate. Doing these things at the first sign of stress can save you from a real meltdown later on.

Anxiety Can Lead to More Serious Conditions

Anxiety that goes unchecked can develop into anxiety disorders. These disorders include social phobias, such as agoraphobia (fear of going out in public), specific phobias (such as fear of dogs or spiders), or obsessive behaviors (such as obsessive hand washing or repeatedly checking door locks or appliance switches).

Women in perimenopause sometimes report the occurrence of panic attacks—overwhelming feelings of intense fear or impending doom that occur suddenly and repeatedly. Symptoms include shortness of breath, choking sensations, heart pounding or palpitations, and the sensation of losing control. If you have episodes that sound like this, talk to your health professional or a counselor. There are effective treatments for panic disorder.

 Alert

> Some of the symptoms of anxiety such as a feeling of doom, shortness of breath, heart palpitations, nausea, and clamminess could also be typically female symptoms of a heart attack. Don't minimize these events, but use them as a chance to rule out physical causes. Discuss them with your medical care provider, and ask whether you should have a cardiac evaluation.

What Is Depression?

The term depression is one you hear frequently. It's not unusual for people to say they're depressed by the weather, their jobs, their haircuts, their prospects for dinner, or the night's television lineup. But there's a world of difference between these passing feelings of disappointment, dissatisfaction, or sadness, and an ongoing state of major depression. For all of the overwrought "depressions" you hear about every day, true depression is a real problem faced by hundreds of thousands of people in our society. According to the Journal of the American Medical Association, between 5 and 10 percent of the U.S. population experiences major depression, and nearly 25 percent of all women will suffer from depression at some point during their lives.

Major depression is an illness that prevents sufferers from working, eating, sleeping, studying, and enjoying a full, normal life and range of moods. Major depression typically results from changes in brain chemistry; therefore, even though it can occur once in a lifetime, many people who suffer from major depression experience it several times.

Menopause and Depression

Many studies have shown that women first experience depression when they're in their twenties, or even younger. And although menopause doesn't automatically signal the onset of depression, women who have suffered from depression earlier in life – or women who have had postpartum depression or even severe premenstrual syndrome (PMS)—are more likely to have recurring depression during perimenopause. Women who have a family history of depression also run more risk of suffering from depression during perimenopause.

Sometimes, depression itself can be a symptom or side effect of some major life event, such as a divorce, the death of a loved one, losing a job, or dealing with a severe or ongoing medical problem—all problems that can occur to women at midlife. But these sorts of event-triggered depressions may pass with time or resolve themselves quickly, without the need for special treatment or therapy. Sometimes, however, these events can lead to depression that deepens into a more systemic, major depression that women are unlikely to overcome without some form of treatment.

Another, less severe, type of depression is known as dysthymia. The symptoms of dysthymia are similar to those of major depression and may be chronic and long term, but they aren't disabling. Finally, bipolar disorder (manic-depressive illness) is another kind of depression. People suffering from a bipolar disorder experience extreme mood shifts that swing wildly between manic highs and depressed lows.

Know the Symptoms of Depression

Though transient feelings of sadness, despair, or a general dissatisfaction with life are common during perimenopause, if these feelings are

The Everything Health Guide to Menopause

long lasting or severe, they could be signaling the onset of depression. Insomnia, fatigue, hot flashes, and other perimenopausal symptoms can trigger minor mood disorders during perimenopause. But major depression goes well beyond the typical reaction to these symptoms and is often the result of a biological or chemical imbalance that requires careful diagnosis and treatment. The National Institute of Mental Health provides a list of common symptoms of depression (though it notes that few people suffer all of them). Here are some of those symptoms:

- Feeling persistently sad, anxious, empty, hopeless, or pessimistic
- A strong sense of impending doom
- A loss of interest in hobbies or activities you once enjoyed (including sex)
- Feeling guilty, worthless, or helpless
- Losing energy and feeling fatigued and slowed down
- Suffering from insomnia, early morning awakening, or oversleeping
- Experiencing a dramatic change in appetite or weight
- Difficulty concentrating, remembering, or making decisions
- Thoughts of suicide and death, or suicide attempts
- Feeling restless and irritable
- Suffering from persistent physical symptoms (headache, pain, digestive disorders) that don't respond to treatment

Essential

If you suffer from low self-esteem, feel overwhelmed by stress, or have a persistently pessimistic attitude toward life, you might be at risk for developing depression. Scientists continue to study the causes of depression to determine whether these types of feelings are an indicator that you're prone to depression, or whether these feelings can actually trigger the illness.

The Causes of Depression

No one cause is at the source of every case of depression, but it usually is associated with a change in the brain's structure or functions. Sometimes a vulnerability to depression is genetically inherited, but depression can be brought on by physical changes resulting from stress, injury, an accident, or a serious emotional event. If an individual feels at the mercy of a disease or illness, he or she can fall into depression. Severe illnesses such as heart attack, stroke, and cancer can lead to depression, as can progressive illnesses such as Parkinson's disease. Financial problems, the death of a loved one, the loss of a job, a parent's illness, the departure of grown children, and other stressful changes to a daily routine also can push people into depression. Even a change of address or an abrupt change in a close circle of friends can trigger the onset of a depression that's been building over time. Finally, hormonal shifts, such as those women experience in pregnancy, perimenopause, and menopause, can also contribute to depression in women.

Considering all these triggers, you easily can see how some women might suffer from depression during perimenopause. Menopause itself doesn't cause depression, but the hormonal changes of perimenopause can join with other natural life events of middle age to contribute to a depressed state.

Take Action

Major depression is an illness, with many options for treatment. The sooner you get help, the more quickly and effectively you can overcome the physical and emotional side effects of this devastating condition. Many women can go through months of emotional turmoil thinking, "It's just a bad day," then "What a bad week," to "This month has been awful," and still believe that they're just feeling temporarily down. Often, these women are taken aback when a friend, spouse, or relative expresses concerns over their moodiness, irritability, or remoteness.

If you or those around you suspect that your emotional behavior may signal a mood disorder, you need to seek a diagnosis and, if necessary, make behavioral changes or begin treatment. Your goal is to get your life back in balance, so you can regain your sense of confidence and purpose.

Alert

As you approach menopause, consider your risks for depression. Do you have a family history of depression? Have you suffered from severe PMS or postpartum depression earlier in your life? If you have a predisposition, don't ignore feelings of depression that arise as you near the age of menopause. Talk to your doctor, therapist, or other health care professional about your concerns early.

Rule Out Medical Causes

Mood swings, depression, and anxiety can all be triggered or made worse by medical problems. Thyroid disorders can sometimes result in depression, as can the use of some medications used to treat high blood pressure. Some weight-loss drugs can trigger a rise in anxiety levels or even panic attacks. Begin by talking with your gynecologist or general practitioner, who can review your medications and health history to uncover any potential medical causes for your mood disorders.

Your doctor or health care provider can also uncover contributing medical conditions, such as insomnia, sleep apnea, or extreme hormonal imbalances, which may contribute to your mood swings. If your doctor uncovers specific medical causes for your condition, he or she can adjust your medication, treat the contributing medical condition, or suggest other specific treatment options to address those issues.

Explore Your Treatment Options

When medical complications have been ruled out, you have several treatment options available to you for diminishing—or even eliminating—your mood disorder symptoms. The option that's best for you is determined, in part, by the severity of your problem and your personal and family medical history.

If you suffer from major depression, your doctor is likely to prescribe an antidepressant medication. Following is a quick list of some of the most commonly prescribed antidepressant and anti-anxiety medications:

- **Selective serotonin reuptake inhibitors (SSRIs),** including fluoxetine, sertraline, paroxetine, and citalopram (marketed as Prozac, Zoloft, Paxil, and Celexa). Though SSRIs can cause depressed sexual response and other side effects in certain individuals, they are non-addictive and work by helping your body make better use of the serotonin it naturally produces. Some of these medications are effective with anxiety as well.

- **Tricyclic antidepressants** such as desipramine, amitriptyline, imipramine and others, have been used for many years to treat depression. While they do have some annoying side effects such as dry mouth, sleepiness, sensitivity to the sun, and low blood pressure, these medications can be very effective in treating depression. Since they interact with many other medications and may change blood sugar levels, you should tell your health provider about all other medications you are on, and any medical conditions you might have before starting these drugs.

- **Anti-anxiety drugs, or anxiolytics**—such as buspirone and alprazolam—can lessen the effects of depression, anxiety, and sleeplessness, and they also can treat the symptoms of PMDD that many perimenopausal women experience as they move closer to menopause. Anxiolytics can have a slightly sedative effect and can be addictive, so many doctors prescribe them for short periods of time only.

 # Fact

Many doctors prescribe antidepressants in combination with hormone therapy for perimenopausal or menopausal women with severe depression. Though hormone therapy is rarely the first-course treatment for depression, it can alleviate symptoms such as hot flashes and insomnia that contribute to depression, and it offers other benefits for some menopausal women.

Psychological counseling—psychotherapy—is a powerful treatment option for women experiencing excess anxiety, stress, or mood disturbance during perimenopause and menopause. Most studies have shown that counseling in conjunction with antidepressant medication offers more long-term and effective results than does a treatment using medication alone. Though you may not experience the benefits of psychotherapy immediately after you begin treatment, its effects can be long lasting and extensive.

The two types of psychotherapy you are most likely to receive for emotional problems associated with perimenopause are interpersonal therapy or cognitive behavioral therapy. Interpersonal therapy explores the relationships in your life and how they contribute to your emotional problems. This type of therapy also teaches you how you may use the strength and support you gain from your relationships to help deal with emotional issues. Cognitive behavioral therapy examines your core thoughts and beliefs and how they determine your actions in response to life. If you have developed a pessimistic or negative attitude toward life, this type of therapy can help you see the world in a more balanced perspective and learn more effective ways of viewing and coping with challenges.

Essential

Learning to be optimistic can have real physical and emotional health benefits. Studies continue to point to the benefits of optimism, including increased feelings of well-being, better immune response, and quicker recovery from injury and disease. Best of all, it can be learned! So even if you aren't rosy by nature, you can learn techniques to have an optimistic outlook that will benefit your physical and emotional health.

Staying "On the Level"

If you are experiencing mild mood disturbances, anxiety, or general but recurring feelings of the blues, you have a number of simple self-treatment options for leveling out the emotional roller-coaster ride.

Give Yourself What You Need

First, give your body and mind healthy amounts of good fuel, activity, and rest. Eat a healthy diet that emphasizes fruit, vegetables, and whole grains and skips high-fat, low-nutrient foods loaded with sugar, salt, and simple carbohydrates. Limiting the amount of caffeine, salt, MSG, and sugar you consume can help your body remain active and alert, rather than jumpy and fatigued. Your physical and emotional health are closely linked, and you can't maintain either with a crummy diet.

Here are some other good guidelines to follow:

- **Eat sensible amounts of food throughout the day.** If you stuff yourself or try to eat your way out of a low mood, you just add to the problem by contributing to weight gain, low self-esteem, and poor body image. Bad nutrition can lead to illness, fatigue, and a host of other problems that can leave you feeling hopeless and depressed. Caring about your body is essential to caring for your mind.

- **Be Active.** Though mood swings, anxiety, and depression can leave you feeling frozen—uninterested in life and incapable of doing anything to participate in it—activity is one of the best ways to lift and stabilize your mood. Physical activity triggers your body to release mood-lifting endorphins, and it gets your heart pumping to circulate oxygenated blood throughout your body. Participating in activities with family and friends can help lighten your mood, broaden your perspective on problems, and help you deal more effectively with issues that threaten your emotional health.

- **Practice meditation or relaxation techniques.** Meditation, relaxation techniques, and mind-body exercises such as yoga and Tai Chi are powerful tools for relieving stress, anxiety, and mild depression (see the section on Mind-Body Exercises in Chapter 5 for more information on these techniques). Fifteen-minute sessions of meditation, deep breathing, or relaxation every morning and evening can help reduce or even eliminate much of the stress and mood-altering emotional upheavals of perimenopause.

- **Get plenty of rest.** Try to establish and maintain a regular sleep schedule, in which you go to sleep and rise at the same times every day—including weekends. Take time to read, listen to music, or soak in a hot tub to relax and prepare yourself for sleep. Don't exercise or eat large amounts of food late in the evening.

 Fact

One study from the University of Washington showed that a simple intervention of a brisk daily twenty-minute walk, more sunlight during the day and less light at night, and taking certain vitamins, could impact women's mood. The program, called LEVITY—for Light, Exercise, and Vitamin Intervention Therapy—improved mood and well-being scores for the women. For details, go to *http://thebodyblues .com/solution.html*.

You Don't Have to Go It Alone

No single treatment option is right—or even effective—for every woman. But any woman suffering from mood disorders should talk with a doctor, counselor, mentor, or other trusted advisor to discuss all appropriate treatments. Depression and other mood disturbances are not a typical by-product of the aging process. A willingness to admit and discuss mood disorders is essential for overcoming them.

Though women are statistically more likely than men are to suffer from depression, they are also more likely to look for help in overcoming issues that affect their emotional health. Your friends, family, coworkers, doctors, minister, or other counselors can help you find ways to put emotional issues to rest, so you can concentrate on becoming healthier, stronger, and more engaged in life as each year passes.

CHAPTER 9

But I'm Still a Woman, Right?—Menopause and Sexuality

THE END OF FERTILITY does not mean the end of sexuality. Despite a culture preoccupied with youth, women can hit their sexual stride in their forties and fifties. Attractiveness does not depend on childbearing, and women find freedom and a depth of sexual maturity after menopause that defies the stereotypes. There is no rule that says sex stops at fifty, and many women find that, in fact, it begins in a whole new way.

Myths and Fears

In the past, it was generally accepted that women lost their desire for sex as they approached menopause, and that the passage through menopause led inevitably toward the eventual death of the libido. Today, most people know that idea is simply untrue and dismiss it as outdated mythology; still, there are physical changes that do affect sexuality and the more familiar you are with them, the better you are able to work with your body to define your sexual self.

Thanks to the burgeoning numbers of women moving into midlife, the discussion, research, and medical information on maturing female sexuality has never been richer. Women can educate themselves about exactly what kinds of physical symptoms and changes may affect their sexuality during menopause and how to maintain optimum sexual health during this time. Being explicit about sexual needs paves the way for a sexual revolution as socially significant as the first one these baby boomers experienced back in the 1960s—an era of the sexually confident, healthy, and vital midlife woman!

Essential

Medical causes of female sexual dysfunction are rarely permanent or untreatable. That's why it's important that any woman experiencing any change in her sexual functions talk to her doctor or health care provider. There is likely to be a treatment or adjustment that will help.

Face It, Don't Fear It

There are some legitimate reasons that sexual desire and activity may slow down during perimenopause. It's best to face them squarely so that they can be addressed. Here are some common reasons women may experience a decline in sexual interest:

- Painful intercourse, resulting from vaginal dryness and atrophy
- Lack of a partner or a partner's declining ability to satisfy
- Feelings of low self-esteem or physical undesirability
- Feeling too tired, too busy, or otherwise preoccupied to enjoy sexual activity

Every woman has unique sexual needs and interests, and many women (and men) have a decreased sexual desire at some point in their lives. But if you find your interest in sex waning—at any age—it's important to understand why. Maintaining and nurturing your sexuality is important for your physical and emotional health. You shouldn't expect to stop enjoying sex as you age.

Listen to Your Sexual Self

Dispelling the myths of sexuality requires being in touch with your authentic sexual self. Your sexuality has evolved with the rest of you, and the entire package has changed dramatically over the past twenty years. Your sexual interests and responses change, too. Sexual techniques you used to enjoy might have lost some—or all—of their appeal over time. As your sexual tastes evolve, you can find totally new and different ways to enjoy sex.

But if you suddenly realize that sex no longer holds any interest for you; or that you don't like your body enough to share it in sexual relations with anyone; or that it's just too painful, awkward, difficult, or otherwise unpleasant to "mess with" sex, ask yourself when—and why—these feelings arose in you. You're too young (at any age) to just walk away from a sexually fulfilling life.

Whatever the culture tells us about sex, staying sexually fulfilled is a normal, reasonable expectation. You deserve and benefit from a healthy, active sex life—whether you have a partner or not. If you aren't enjoying (or even thinking about) sex, you have many options for regaining your sexual enjoyment—whether that involves exploring new sexual techniques, examining your attitudes about sexuality, or investigating possible medical causes for your diminishing sexual interests or abilities.

 Fact

A landmark 1986 study by Masters and Johnson (Sex and Aging—Expectations and Reality) found that women can remain sexually active their entire lives with no decline in orgasmic potential, and may even become more orgasmic. The study also found that normal changes of sexual response and aging don't equate to decreased sexual functioning.

Checking Your Sexual Attitude

Your attitudes about sex and your own sexuality today are greatly influenced by the attitudes you had about these issues when you were younger. If you enjoyed sex and expected to be sexually satisfied when you were thirty, you're more likely to continue to enjoy sex as you move through your fifties and beyond. Nevertheless, some women report a declining interest in sex after menopause, and most experts agree that changes in attitude can play a big role in that shift.

Beyond the Physical Factor

A woman's psychological and emotional state can trigger many of the physical symptoms associated with aging sexuality. When a woman has low self-esteem or a poor body image, for example, she may not respond as well to stimulation. Anxiety, sleeplessness, and hot flashes can interfere with your ability to anticipate or enjoy sex. Decreased sexual activity itself can lead to diminished sexual desire, pleasure, and response. A woman with a sexually dysfunctional partner—or no partner at all—can be at risk of losing her own sexual health as a result.

You probably know that your most important responses to sexual stimulation take place in your brain. Perimenopause and natural menopause are transitions associated with aging, and if self-esteem suffers as a result of aging, sexual desire may suffer, too. Our bodies change during perimenopause; that, too, is an undeniable fact. The degree of that change varies, of course, and we have many tools to help maintain our physical health and vitality as we grow older. But women who combat weight gain, fatigue, depression, and feelings of isolation during perimenopause are at risk for suffering from flagging sexual desire as well.

It's Not Just about You

Our partners—male or female—are changing, too. Two women going through perimenopause at the same time may experience a multitude of sexual issues as they try to maintain their sexual closeness as each rides her own roller coaster of menopausal symptoms. Men can experience a loss of sexual potency and desire as they age, and that can have a direct impact on the sexual confidence and health of their partners. If a sexual partner seems uninterested in sex or unable to sustain an erection or become aroused, it's easy for the other partner to feel inadequate, undesirable, and definitely unsexy. And it is devastating to a sense of self if your partner separates from you or divorces you, leaving you to feel bereft and inadequate.

Some women find that even in the face of losses, perimenopause is an opportunity to improve their sex lives. These major changes challenge women to reassess their lives, their relationships, and their attitudes toward living. You have a wide variety of physical and psychological tools available to you to help take your sexuality to new heights as your body enjoys sex for reasons that have nothing to do with reproduction.

The Physical Impact of Changing Hormones

Attitude is one thing, but there is no denying that as hormones change, so does your body. What physical symptoms and changes can interfere with sexual desire and pleasure as menopause approaches? Here are the most common:

- Vaginal dryness
- Pain during penetration
- Reduced response to clitoral stimulation and other sexual stimuli

Some of these changes are normal parts of the aging process and don't represent alarming signals that sexual life is drawing to a close. Women (and men, for that matter) typically experience a slowdown in their biologic sexual response. Women may take longer to become aroused, for example, and some women report that they have fewer orgasmic contractions and shorter orgasms in general. These changes may mean that lovemaking takes on a new schedule or some new practices—changes that can benefit lovemaking at any age. Other physical changes are transient and treatable, either with medical hormonal therapies or nonhormonal, natural techniques.

But a maturing woman can undergo a number of physical and medical events that can trigger the symptoms and conditions of flagging sexual health, as well. These events include:

- Illnesses, both physical and emotional, including (but not limited to) cardiac problems, hypertension, cancer, bladder disease, depression, and arthritis
- Medications used to treat any of the above illnesses, including some blood pressure medications, antidepressants, tranquilizers, and antihistamines
- Medical treatments, such as radiation therapy, chemotherapy, or surgery

Don't get the impression that if you take blood pressure medication or undergo surgery that you're embarking on a life of sexual abstinence. Sexual dysfunction resulting from illness or long-term treatments such as chemotherapy can pass as the illness and treatment side effects fade. A number of alternative medications can replace those that create sexual problems.

Hormones and Sexuality

Hormones—especially estrogen—play an important role in your body's sexual response. Estrogen helps to nourish all of your body's tissues, including your vagina, vulva, and urethra. Estrogen also helps keep the clitoris well nourished and responsive; with less estrogen, the clitoris can lose some of its ability to respond to touch.

As your vaginal wall becomes thinner and drier, your vagina can become shorter, narrower, and less elastic. This is called vaginal atrophy and when it becomes severe, sex can be quite painful. Lack of lubrication and vaginal walls that just won't give can make sex less appealing—to both you and your partner.

A lack of estrogen will also result in a change in the normal vaginal pH and lower levels of lactobacillus, the normal bacteria that helps ward off most vaginal infections in reproductive age women. Thus, if your vagina goes through marked changes in pH levels, you may find that you're more susceptible to vaginal infections. These infections can make your vagina feel raw and irritated, create abnormal vaginal discharge, and make sexual intercourse a painful, burning experience. Estrogen therapy can improve vaginal secretions and tone. To reduce the risks from oral or transdermal (also called "the estrogen patch") estrogen therapy, you might want to consider getting estrogen from a vaginal cream. This cream may take a few months to reverse the changes in the vagina, especially if you have been without any estrogen for a long time. But it is absorbed only locally (in the vaginal area), and does not carry the risks of systemic estrogen.

Hormones play another critical role in strengthening or diminishing the libido; the sex hormones—estrogen and progesterone—contribute to mood. If you grow anxious, depressed, irritable, or exhausted as a result of hormone deficiencies, your sex life can suffer.

Fact

> Testosterone treatment for women with marked decrease in sexual desire is controversial. Some studies seem to show that women can benefit from testosterone to renew their sex drive. But the FDA has not yet approved these treatments and appropriate dosages are not yet clear. The side effects of lowering your "good" cholesterol, acne, and excess body hair can also be undesirable.

Overcoming Physical Barriers

Although you can't postpone menopause or the effects of aging indefinitely, you don't have to let some of the physical symptoms of menopause prevent you from remaining sexually active. Your doctor can recommend treatment options, exercise, dietary or medication changes, or other therapeutic solutions that can lessen or even resolve your physical barriers to an enjoyable sex life. And, as with all aspects of your health care, you may be able to improve your sexual health through some changes in your lifestyle choices.

The same stresses, habits, and substances that damage other aspects of your health can limit your desire and ability to enjoy sex, as well. Here are some basics for maintaining your sexual fitness:

- **Eat right and exercise regularly.** Nutrition and exercise are just as important for sexual health as for general physical and emotional health. Regular aerobic, weight-bearing, and stretching exercises keep your body feeling active and alive. When your body is strong and fit, you're more energetic and you take a greater interest in all aspects of your life—including sex.
- **Rest and manage stress.** If your daily routine is too overwhelming to allow you to enjoy an active sex life, it's probably damaging your health in other ways. Stress can lead to headaches, indigestion, muscle pain, depression, and—not surprisingly— a diminished desire for and response to sexual activity. Learn

what's causing your stress, then do what you can to avoid the stressors.

- **Cut down on alcohol and stop smoking.** Most medical experts agree that one or two alcoholic drinks a day aren't bad for your health (unless you have conditions or are taking medication that precludes the use of any alcohol). But drinking too much alcohol can lead to depression, weight gain, and—in some cases—an increased stress response. Smoking fuels stress, as well, and it saps your body of strength and energy. All of these effects can erode your interest in sexual activity and dampen your response to sexual stimulation.

Maintaining Your Sexual Health

It's good to note that nearly every symptom or problem that affects your sexual health is treatable, reversible, or even avoidable. But, as with any area of your health maintenance, you can't count on someone else—your doctor, minister, therapist, or partner—to protect and manage your sexual health. That job is yours.

Essential

A multivitamin-mineral supplement may be an easy and inexpensive way to promote your sexuality—and your general health. Vitamin E has been shown in some studies to increase sexual desire, and zinc may help foster sexual arousal (oysters are high in zinc). Selenium is another mineral that is the subject of ongoing studies of sexuality.

If you, like the vast majority of men and women in this country, intend to remain sexually active throughout a long and healthy life, what can you do to ensure that you maintain your sexual health through the years ahead? For starters, you have four very basic tools at your disposal for monitoring and maintaining your sexual health:

- Monitor your sexual health and pay attention to changes in your sexual responses and feelings.
- Maintain an open dialog with your health care professional about sexual problems and solutions.
- Protect yourself from pregnancy and sexually transmitted disease while still in perimenopause.

Vaginal Health

Frankly stated, an active fulfilling sexuality requires a healthy vagina. Your vagina is maturing along with the rest of your body, and it's worth your while to pay some special attention to caring for this sensitive (and vital) part of your body. Don't worry—you don't need a special course in maintenance and repair to keep this part of your sexual being in order. Some very simple techniques and common-sense practices can help you maintain your vaginal health.

First, if your sexual life involves new partners, always practice safe sex. This isn't the 1960s, and casual unprotected sex with strangers never again will be in fashion. Don't count on your judgment or gut reaction to determine whether or not someone's infected with human immunodeficiency virus (HIV) or other sexually transmitted diseases (STDs). Assume that they are—no matter who they are—and don't allow a sexual partner's semen, blood, or other body fluids to come in contact with your vagina, anus, or mouth. Your vaginal tissues are becoming thinner and easier to tear, and your immune system might be stressed by shifting hormone levels. That puts you more at risk than ever for contracting a sexually transmitted disease. Talk to your partner about his or her sexual history, use condoms, and get blood tests. Safe sex practices may not seem sexy, but they're basic to survival.

Next, take steps to reduce vaginal dryness. Your vaginal secretions diminish along with your estrogen level, which can contribute to dry, inflexible vaginal tissues and painful intercourse. Your vagina's pH balance will shift with your hormone levels, too, and that can contribute to increased irritation and bacterial infections. Estrogen therapy is one way to combat vaginal dryness, but it's not the only method for keeping vaginal tissues moist and pliant.

Over-the-counter vaginal moisturizers such as Astroglide, K-Y Jelly, and Vagisil Moisturizer can help fight off dryness. (Ask your doctor or pharmacist for other vaginal moisturizing products.) Avoid vaginal deodorizers and deodorized products, scented toilet tissues, and chemical-laden bath soaps and soaks. Perfumes and chemicals can further upset the pH balance in your vagina and contribute to local irritation and dryness. Water hydrates all of your cells; drink between thirty-two and sixty-four ounces every day to keep your skin, hair, bones, and other body tissues fully moisturized.

 Alert

Ten percent of new HIV/AIDS cases are in people over fifty. Because older people are not routinely tested for HIV and are not as familiar with how it spreads, they are at higher risk for having undiagnosed cases. They may mistake symptoms for the aches of getting older and are often embarrassed to discuss this with their medical provider. Use safe sex practices with any new partners, and ask your partners about their HIV status.

Improve Sexual Response with the Kegel Exercise

You've probably heard of the Kegel exercise; many women use them to return the strength and condition of their vaginal muscles after childbirth. Other women use the Kegel exercise to improve their ability to control stress incontinence. Kegel exercise has also been shown to offer women another important benefit: Strengthening vaginal muscles can increase sexual health and pleasure.

The exercises strengthen the pelvic floor muscles that extend from the pubic bone to the tailbone and surround your vaginal opening and the opening to your urinary tract. Strengthening these muscles enables you to contract your vaginal opening, increasing the amount and intensity of the contact between your vagina and your partner's penis. Kegel exercise also increases the blood flow to (and the sensitivity of) your genital area. Practicing them regularly can increase the physical sensations of intercourse, making sex more pleasurable for both you and your partner.

 Fact

Obstetrician/gynecologist Arnold Kegel developed the exercise named for him in the mid-1940s as a non-surgical solution for his patients who were battling incontinence. He later realized that the exercises helped new mothers recover from the physical effects of labor and vaginal childbirth. Today, many women do the Kegel exercise to make their vaginal muscles stronger and more resilient in preparation for childbirth.

You can find your vaginal muscles the next time you urinate. When you begin urinating, squeeze your muscles to stop the flow. Try to start and stop the flow several times, in the same sitting. The muscles you're contracting are those of your pelvic floor musculature—the same set of muscles that you exercise with the Kegel exercise. Once you learn to identify and contract that muscle, you can do your exercises anywhere. (And once you've identified them, don't use them to stop your urine anymore – that can be bad for your bladder.) Contract the pelvic floor muscle and hold it for a count of five. Breathe normally and repeat the contraction, hold, and release ten times. Do this exercise every day—do a dozen repetitions when you're sitting and waiting for a red light to change, or when you're on hold for a phone call. After a month or two of practice, you should notice that you have more control over your bladder and some improved sensation during sexual activity (even masturbation).

Talk about S-E-X

As your sexuality matures with you, you might experience any or all of the problems or issues discussed in this chapter. And, in most cases, you may need to talk to a medical professional, therapist, or other counselor or consultant to find the best resolution for those problems. If you aren't comfortable discussing medical or emotional aspects of your sexuality or sexual health, that discomfort can make your situation seem even more frustrating and hopeless. Your ability to talk about issues—ranging from painful intercourse to a lack of response to stimulation—is crucial to establish a trusting relationship with your health care provider, and to become comfortable discussing your sexual health with that person.

Begin by talking to the health care professional or counselor you trust most. If that person can't provide the professional assistance you need, he or she can refer you to the appropriate source for that help.

Relationships and Menopause

As indicated in AARP's Sexuality at Midlife and Beyond study, the majority of people over forty-five think that sexuality is an important part of relationships. It was also clear in this study that staying physically and emotionally healthy was critical in sustaining a satisfying marriage or partnership.

If you are in a committed relationship as you near midlife, the chances are good that your partner in that relationship is aging, too. His or her sexual performance and desire may be suffering as much—or even more—than your own. If you and your partner experience a decline in sexual intimacy, talk about it.

Essential

One of the findings of the AARP update to their sexuality study was that women reported greater sexual satisfaction when their male partners used medications for erectile dysfunction. Women are responding to their partners' renewed enthusiasm, with the result that both partners feel more eager and satisfied.

If your partner is suffering from physical problems that are affecting his or her sexual performance, talking with a doctor is the next step. A general practitioner or gynecologist may decide to refer you to a sex therapist, if your condition warrants that treatment. Keep an open mind and follow your doctor's recommendations. Again, maintaining the health of your sexual relationship is an important part of remaining healthy and happy together.

Enhancing Your Sexual Experience

You may find that your lovemaking simply needs some new life. Take this opportunity to enjoy a second "first romance" with your partner. Learn to touch each other again and take pleasure in your physical contact; take baths and showers together and spend more time in touching and foreplay during lovemaking. Let your partner know what feels good to you and find out what he or she enjoys most, and explore your fantasies. You might surprise each other—you being confident, your partner being responsive to your confidence. Give it a whirl.

Suggestions for Your Sexual Self—This Could Be Fun!

If you lead a hectic life, filled with the responsibilities of work, home, and family, there's little time to think about yourself—your body, your mind, your pleasure. As your body begins to change with age, you may begin to think of it as an adversary instead of an ally. Something you've always depended on (though you may not have lavished much attention on it) that's letting you down just when you need it most. Many women simply lose touch with their physicality, choosing to ignore their physical condition and respond in the out-of-sight-out-of-mind approach we all know so well.

Enjoying Your Body

The truth is that your body matters. All of this book's recommendations for exercise, health care, regular checkups, relaxation techniques, hair and skin treatments, and good diet are aimed at the important goal of taking care of your body so you can enjoy it. By feeling confident and at ease about your body, you're more likely to enjoy the pleasures of its sexual response. Learn to include your sexuality in your identity;

humans are sexual beings, and sexual enjoyment is good for the body, mind, and spirit.

Explore your sexual interests and fantasies. Your sexual orientation, desires, and needs are assets, not liabilities. Many doctors and sex therapists encourage their patients to masturbate to increase their ability to respond to sexual stimulation and to combat stress and anxiety.

Reach out for more information on sexual response. Visit your local bookstore, where you can find many self-help books on improving your sexual response. Even reading a steamy novel can help you to become aroused. Or rent a film with some love scenes featuring a favorite movie star. You don't have to turn to pornography, just allow yourself to explore and enjoy the sexual arousal you might normally hold back.

 # Fact

Exercise offers a number of benefits for women at any age, but did you know that it could give you a real sexual boost? Some studies have shown that people who practice some form of regular exercise achieve orgasm more easily than do people who don't exercise at all.

Be Creative

Many women expect spontaneous bursts of admiration from their partners, even if they haven't been demonstrating much interest in their body or their sexuality lately. Take some time to do the things that will make you look and feel more beautiful. Get a new haircut or have a facial. Stop by the cosmetics counter at your local department store and ask for some ideas for revitalizing your appearance. When you look better, you feel more sexually appealing.

Would a new nightgown make you feel sexier? If you've grown self-conscious about your midlife physique, wearing a flattering negligee during lovemaking can help you feel more confident and relaxed. Silky, flattering lingerie comes in a variety of styles and sizes, so visit a lingerie store to check out your options. And while you're there, try some of the new bust-shaping brassieres. Many women in midlife have cleavage for the first time, so why not take advantage of it?

Ĺ, Essential

As he ages, your male partner may need more stimulation in order to achieve an erection. As you're learning to enjoy your sexuality more, don't forget to pay attention to your partner's needs. Many couples find that as their sexual relationship matures they draw increasing pleasure from the non-intercourse parts of their lovemaking, and use their hands and mouths more frequently during sex.

Setting the mood is all-important for revitalizing your lovemaking. Lower the lights, burn some aromatic candles, and play some soft, sensual music. Now is the time to relax and explore sensual pleasures. Put away the sweatpants and dress for dinner—if you're dining at home, why not try a "French maid" costume? Use your imagination and have fun with sex. Be creative, experiment, and be open with your partner about your feelings and responses to whatever you experience together.

Don't Forget about Birth Control

There's an old joke: What's the best birth control for people over fifty? Answer: Nudity. Not only is this obviously a bit psychologically discouraging, it's also false. Remember, until you have gone for twelve months without a period or until your doctor or health care provider has run appropriate blood tests to determine the levels of hormones your body is producing, you could ovulate and, therefore, become pregnant after sexual activity. Many women stop using birth control after they've missed four or five periods and feel that they're no longer fertile. That's a mistake; a surprise pregnancy in your mid-forties can be a tremendous problem for both you and your partner. Again, be smart, and use contraceptives for a year after your last period.

Chapter 10

A Partner on the Path— Choosing a Health Provider

IN AN AGE OF HMOS, PPOs, and a never-ending list of traditional and alternative health care provider options, few women go through their adult lives with a single practitioner. The increased mobility of modern life does away with the lifetime family doctor, too. That's why it's important for every woman to become an active member of her health care "plan" by working closely with her primary care provider.

Do You Have the Provider You Need Now?
The chance that you'll see the same health care professional at age fifty that you saw at age twenty is very low. With the ever-changing parade of health care workers we see over the course of our lives, it's easy to think of them as interchangeable cogs in the vast machine of our professional health care maintenance. But that's a dangerous attitude to have toward the people responsible for helping you live a long, healthy life.

Your Changing Needs
Your choice of a health care professional must always meet certain qualifications in training and ability. But when you're approaching menopause, you require some special qualities in a health care provider. If you have been a passive patient up to this point, now's the time to get involved in ensuring your good health throughout menopause—and beyond.

Does Your Provider Understand Your Menopause?
During perimenopause and menopause, your health care needs differ from those when you were younger. You may need diagnosis and treatment of emotional as well as physical symptoms. And you certainly

will need the medical advice of someone who is up-to-date on medical advancements in menopause symptoms and treatment, knowledge-able about a range of treatment options, and willing and able to discuss those options with you. Even if you've been pretty casual about health care during your twenties, thirties, and early forties, your health care actions and choices now can determine the quality of the rest of your life.

You may have a great health care provider right now, or you may want to begin your search for the doctor who's right for you. In either case, now is the time to evaluate what you want and need in a health care provider and to make sure that you have the man or woman who fulfills that role.

Question

Can't my primary care physician handle my health care during menopause?

If both you and your primary care provider (PCP) are comfortable with that arrangement, there's no reason for you to see a specialist during menopause. If you have severe or unusual symptoms, how-ever, your PCP is likely to refer you to a specialist for diagnosis and treatment. Talk to your PCP about his or her recommendations for your health care during menopause.

Personal Qualities of Your Health Care Provider

When you're choosing a health care provider to give you appropriate medical oversight and guidance, you need to consider a number of qualities. Medical or professional licensing and board certification are a must. But beyond that, what qualities matter most to you in a health care professional? Maybe up to this point, you've been very comfortable with the gruff, no-nonsense doctor who tells you, "This is what you need to do, now go do it," and moves on. Now, however, you may want a doctor who's willing to listen to your fears, questions, and concerns, and who will encourage you to take an active role in managing your health care.

Or maybe you've been perfectly content with the catch-as-catch-can variability of health care service provided by a large local clinic, but now you want to establish a strong relationship with a doctor and start getting more personalized, in-depth care, testing, and treatment. How do you decide what you need your doctor to do—or be?

Which Provider Fits You?

The first step in choosing the right health care provider for your menopause journey is to determine what kind of person you want to work with.

Ask yourself these questions:

- **Do you prefer to see a male or a female health care professional?** You're going to need to be comfortable with this person, so you need to decide if gender plays a role in your willingness to discuss symptoms, lifestyle factors, and treatment alternatives. If you'll feel reluctant to be totally open and honest with a health care provider because of his or her gender, this may not be the time to try to break down those barriers.
- **Do you want a medical "boss" who will dispense advice and guidance without requesting your input regarding treatment options?** Or would you prefer someone who is open to the patient-as-partner approach to health care? There's nothing wrong with expecting your health care provider to suggest specific treatment options—as long as that person is fully trained and has a complete understanding of your medical background and family history. If, on the other hand, you want to discuss and choose from a range of options, you need to be certain that your health care provider is willing to discuss those options with you and support your decision with good follow-through treatment.
- **Do you care about the age of your health care provider?** Again, it's important that you feel comfortable so that you can openly discuss your health and lifestyle issues and will be confident in the decisions and recommendations that you're offered.

L. Essential

> While personal qualities don't determine a health care profession-
> al's skills or training, they may influence the way you work with that
> person. In the end, you might choose someone who doesn't fit your
> optimum personality profile, but acknowledging your preferences
> can help you form a strong working relationship with any health
> care professional.

It's Your Choice

If you give some time to thinking about the sort of care provider who can help you through the menopausal transition, you will have a better chance of finding the right person. You will want someone with whom you are comfortable and who can answer your questions and provide safe, competent care. The more comfortable you are with this person, the more likely you are to discuss your symptoms and concerns. Even if he or she is not an expert in gynecology, a provider who can answer your questions and can refer you when an issue is beyond his or her expertise may be the right provider for you.

Professional Qualifications

Personal qualities aside, the most important factor in your choice of a health care provider should be professional training. When you're choosing medical care specifically for your treatment during meno-pause, you need first to decide what kind of special training you want your caregiver to have. If you want someone with specialization beyond that of a family practitioner, you can choose from among several types of traditional and nontraditional health care providers.

Traditional Health Care Providers

You may be the sort of person who feels most comfortable with a traditional provider, or you may live in a city or town where that is the only choice available to you. Within the realm of traditional medicine, here are some of your choices:

- An obstetrician/gynecologist (ob/gyn) is specially trained in prenatal care for expectant mothers and the delivery of babies (the obstetrician part) and care of women's reproductive health from menarche to menopause and beyond (the gynecologist services). These physicians can provide long-term treatment for women at any development stage or age. You can also choose an ob/gyn with a specialization in menopause. These specialists remain up-to-date on menopause symptoms, testing, and treatment methods, and new developments in the use of menopausal hormone therapies (MHT).

- A reproductive endocrinologist is a doctor who specializes in hormone imbalances and infertility. Since these physicians focus on reproductive hormones, they are familiar with MHT and other treatments and issues that impact menopausal women. Some of these physicians deal strictly with infertility issues, so check before you make the appointment.

- A nurse practitioner is a registered nurse (R.N.) who has advanced training and can perform physical examinations, diagnose and treat illnesses and injuries, prescribe medication, and provide other health care functions. A women's health nurse practitioner (W.H.N.P.) has special training in the area of women's health. Recent studies have shown that many people of both sexes are choosing nurse practitioners as primary health care providers, citing satisfaction with such factors as how much time they spend discussing health issues and how available they are to their patients.

- Naturopaths are healthcare providers who work with the body's natural ability to heal itself and may employ many approaches to your menopausal symptoms including diet changes, nutritional supplements, herbal medicine, acupuncture or Chinese medicine, hydrotherapy, massage, joint manipulation, and/or lifestyle counseling.

Complementary/Alternative Care Providers

Complementary and alternative medicine (CAM) is big business in the United States. According to the National Center for Complementary and Alternative Healthcare (NCCAM), a branch of the National Institutes of Health (NIH), 36 percent of adults in the United States use some form of CAM. If you consider megavitamin therapy and prayer specifically for health reasons, that number rises to 62 percent. Many women turn to alternative health care techniques during menopause; here are some of the types of health care providers they choose:

- **Herbalists** prescribe herbal supplements and treatments to combat symptoms of menopause. Herbal remedies are growing in popularity in Western cultures, and herbalists are trained to help determine the best types, amounts, and delivery mechanisms for herbal treatment of menopause symptoms.
- **Homeopaths** offer a type of medical treatment that operates on the principle that like cures like. Homeopaths prescribe small doses of substances that, if not diluted, would actually make symptoms worse; homeopathic prescription amounts are based on the severity of symptoms, rather than the age and weight of the patient.
- **Acupuncturists** use a 2,000-year-old treatment technique that involves rotating fine, sterilized needles into the patient's skin to bring about a therapeutic response. Many women in menopause turn to acupuncture for relief of such symptoms as headache, hot flashes, anxiety, insomnia, and fatigue.

 Alert

"Natural" doesn't necessarily mean "safe." Though you can purchase many over-the-counter herbal supplements for relief of menopausal symptoms, you need to be careful. Many plants and herbs deliver significant doses of estrogen or interact with other supplements and prescription drugs. Check with your doctor or health care provider before embarking on any type of alternative treatment.

For a more complete discussion of alternative treatments for symptoms of menopause, see Chapter 12. Many women use alternative medicine techniques to combat symptoms of menopause in conjunction with traditional medical health care. If you're interested in exploring both traditional and alternative medical approaches to treating your menopause symptoms, make sure any health care provider you choose is open to helping you as you pursue this approach.

Finding the Right Fit

There are many ways to look for a health provider whose qualifications match your needs. Ideally, you will explore your options early in your menopausal process. You can approach your search for a suitable care provider as a research project.

Where to Start

Finding a new health care provider can seem mysterious or overwhelming. But if you've decided you want someone who understands menopause, you have some choices in approach. Here are just a few ways you can locate a health care provider:

- **Ask your primary healthcare provider or family physician.** He or she may know the qualified individuals in your area, and since this person knows your style and personality, he or she may be able to match you with someone that's right for you.
- **Ask your family and friends.** Though the practitioner that's best for them may not be the one for you, the women you know can give you an inside perspective on their health care providers. Coworkers may also be able to suggest a physician who is close to your workplace or associated with a nearby hospital. And since your coworkers may be on the same insurance plan that you have, they might be able to help you anticipate—or even avoid—problems with insurance filing.
- **Visit the consumer section of the North American Menopause Society (NAMS) Web site** at *www.menopause.org* to download a list of health care providers registered with the Society as

menopause specialists. The listing indicates licensing and location to help you narrow your search in these key areas.

- **Call reputable medical clinics in your area** to find out if their services include a menopause clinic or specialists.
- **Check with your insurance provider to see if it offers a list of doctors and therapists with menopause specialties.** Most health insurance companies have Web sites listing physicians in your area or affiliated with major hospitals.
- **Go online.** You can search for menopause specialists in your area using any of the major search engines such as Google, Yahoo!, Search.msn, Excite, Dogpile, and others.

Do Your Homework

When you've narrowed the list of potential health care providers, you can explore each health care provider's operation to find out how well it meshes with your needs and preferences. Follow a few practical guidelines for screening health care provider candidates:

- Call the office, and pay attention to the details of your experience. Is the office big and busy or small and personal? Are you immediately put on hold, and if so, how long do you wait? Can the receptionist answer your questions or put you in contact with someone who can? What are the office hours? How long will it take for you to get an appointment? What's the length of an average office visit? You want to make sure you have adequate time with the doctor or practitioner during your visit. Can patients get responses to questions over the telephone or through e-mail? If so, who returns those calls or e-mails?
- Find out what kinds of insurance the office accepts, and how insurance billing is handled. You'll also want to check with your insurance provider to be certain that any alternative or specialty treatment you receive is covered before accepting any potentially expensive testing or treatment plan.
- Try to schedule an information visit with the doctor or practitioner and use that visit to assess: the condition of the office, the helpfulness of the staff, and your impression of the health

care provider. If the doctor or practitioner doesn't limit his or her practice to menopause (and most don't), find out approximately what percentage of the patient load involves menopause treatment.

- Find out if the practice has a person—such as an office manager or assistant to the primary health care provider—who can answer your questions and help you get the service you need when the doctor or practitioner is busy or away from the office. Some offices have a registered nurse who performs this function, while others use a medical assistant or a patient services coordinator with extensive medical knowledge and training. The title isn't as important as this individual's willingness and ability to help you resolve issues that might come up.

Your prescreening efforts are worth the time and effort you invest in them. The health care provider you choose will be an important part of your life for several years to come. Choosing the provider who works best for you can make all of your health care decisions easier and help ensure that you get the best available care, advice, and guidance.

 # Fact

> Your health care provider has a big impact on the decisions you make about therapies and treatment. In one study by a medical researcher from the Harvard Medical School, 96 percent of women in an HMO who had received an initial prescription for MHT cited their doctor's opinion as critical to their decision to pursue that treatment option.

Talk with Your Doctor

Finding a great doctor or other health care provider is only half of the picture. You are the other half. You need to be an active, informed, involved partner in your health care program. Reading this book indicates that you understand the importance of becoming well informed about menopause issues, symptoms, and treatment options. Use the information you find here (and in the recommended resources listed in Appendix C) to decide what kinds of questions and options you want to explore. The following sections discuss some simple ways you can prepare to be a good collaborator who brings out the best in her good provider.

Taking Charge—Start with Honesty

If you're seeing a doctor or practitioner about issues related to menopause, you aren't a kid anymore. As obvious as that seems, it's important that you drop a lot of the passive techniques you may have developed when dealing with doctors in your youth. Do your health care provider a favor, and approach your consultation as an exchange of information— not a tell-me-what-to-do-and-I'll-leave event.

During your initial office visit, the doctor or practitioner will ask you questions about your individual and family health histories. As a rule, you'll need to report on any personal and family history of blood clots, heart disease, breast cancer, osteoporosis, and other selected conditions. Your doctor or practitioner will also ask you about your current medications—both over-the-counter and prescription drugs—as well as your use of alcohol, recreational drugs, and tobacco. You're not running for class president here, so don't attempt to whitewash the facts by presenting yourself as you think you should be. If you drink or smoke, say so. And don't forget that over-the-counter medications such as pain relievers, vitamins, minerals, and nutritional supplements count; report any substances you regularly consume, so your doctor or practitioner can be aware of them when he or she prescribes treatment.

 Alert

When you're visiting your menopause specialist, tell it like it is— don't exaggerate or downplay the symptoms you've experienced. Your caregiver needs to understand the full range and severity of your symptoms. You can't get the best treatment if you aren't completely honest.

During your first visit, remember to mention all symptoms you've been experiencing—both emotional and physical. If your periods have become irregular in any way, report the irregularities. (Take your menstrual calendar to the visit.) Mood swings and depression are important indicators of your current health, as is any change in your interest in sex. If you're suffering from periodic involuntary urine release, report that and explain the conditions. Take a written list of symptoms, questions, and concerns with you to your visit, and write down the answers.

🔲 Essential

If you've been keeping a menstruation journal or menstrual calendar (see Appendix B), take it to your initial visit with your menopause specialist. Your doctor can gain valuable information about your current condition by reviewing even a two- or three-month history of your symptoms. Add to your calendar any symptoms that seem to run in cycles, such as headaches, water retention, or unusual pelvic pain.

Ask for What You Need

Before you leave the office, make sure you understand all of the information you've received during your visit. If you need further explanation, ask for it. If your doctor or practitioner is using terms you don't understand, ask for a translation. Asking for clarification immediately is preferable to calling the office after you've returned home to admit that you didn't understand something you were told. Many doctors' offices also have helpful brochures describing various aspects of menopause, so feel free to ask.

Finally, discuss all treatment options that interest you, regardless of the medical specialization of the health care provider you've chosen. If you're interested in pursuing a combination approach to managing symptoms of menopause, explore whether this doctor or practitioner is open to that approach. If you are looking for relief from specific symptoms, such as incontinence or insomnia, say so and ask if any recommended treatment options specifically address those symptoms. If you think you may want certain tests that the doctor hasn't actually offered, speak up. If you have insurance coverage issues, bring this up as well. The more you understand about the details and goals of treatment options, the better able you'll be to decide which plan is right for you (and the more likely you'll be to follow the plan as recommended).

Take an Active Role

In order for any therapy to be effective, you must be committed to following it—as directed—for as long as is necessary to gauge its results and effectiveness. Being an active partner in your treatment plan involves carefully monitoring your response to therapeutic drugs and treatments, and keeping your health care provider(s) informed of your progress. If you have a negative reaction to drugs or other treatment options, report it. You could be experiencing normal adjustment reactions or you could be embarking on a plan that simply doesn't match your body chemistry, lifestyle, or biological and physiological makeup. You won't know what's wrong unless you report the reaction to your doctor or practitioner.

You Are Your Own Case Manager

If you are using a combination of treatment options, make sure that you coordinate all of them with your primary caregiver. Maybe you've heard about the benefits of using biofeedback-assisted behavioral training to control urine discharge, and you'd like to explore that option. Before you contact a psychologist, physical therapist, or clinician to schedule a biofeedback session, talk to your menopause specialist about the process, to make sure biofeedback won't conflict with other treatment plans you're pursuing. Seeking a second opinion is fine, and often is a good idea, but remember to reflect on all the options you have been offered, and consult the specialist you feel most comfortable with about combining therapies.

When the Plan Isn't Working

Finally, don't remain passively disappointed with your treatment. If you feel unhappy with the health care you're receiving, share that. Your doctor, practitioner, or therapist can't correct a problem that he or she doesn't know about. If you're unhappy with the progress of your symptom-relief treatment, discuss your concerns with your menopause specialist. If you feel that your doctor or practitioner is not responding to your questions and concerns, give him or her an opportunity to discuss your feelings. Although you want to build and maintain a respectful relationship with your caregiver, choose honesty over diplomacy. Be very specific and open as you state your concerns, and listen carefully to your caregiver's response. If you can't resolve your differences, this may not be the right health care partner.

Instructions for putting together your post-forty health management plan appear in Appendix D. But for now, it's important to remember that active, involved follow-through is a critical component of any treatment and lifestyle plan you adopt.

 Alert

Don't judge the quality of your menopause specialist by how often that person agrees with you. You want a health care provider who'll help you pursue treatment that's effective and safe. Find someone you can trust, then discuss your concerns and ideas with an open mind, and—if necessary—seek a second or third opinion.

Listen Up, Speak Up, Be Honest

Throughout this chapter, you're reminded that you carry a big part of the responsibility for making sure that you get the best possible health care. When you've chosen a health care provider who meets your needs and fits your own list of qualifications, you still don't get to sit back and enjoy the ride. To make sure that you help your health care provider give you the best advice and treatment options during your transition through perimenopause, remember the following important guidelines:

- Listen to the information your health care provider gives you. When you ask a question, take notes of the response if necessary; don't assume that you already know what your caregiver is going to say. Just listen carefully, and ask further questions, if necessary.

- Ask questions, voice concerns, report problems, and discuss options; your caregiver depends upon your active feedback.
- Be honest. You must be honest in your communications with your health care provider. Many people think that they'll annoy their doctor or health care provider by asking too many questions or by discussing issues that they don't fully understand or agree with.

Most doctors and other health care providers find it much more challenging to deal with patients who act as though they're okay with a plan or fully understand a treatment option, when that isn't really the case. You can't have a good health care experience if you don't communicate openly and honestly with your health care provider.

CHAPTER 11

Deciding Whether Hormone Therapy Is Right for You

THE DECISION TO USE ESTROGEN and other hormones to treat symptoms during perimenopause has always been a struggle for women. Comparing health risks with the benefits of hormone therapy has become even more confusing in recent years with the reporting of the Women's Health Initiative (WHI) study and its unexpected results. This chapter will sort out some of the elements of hormone therapy so that you can make the best decision for your unique set of risks and concerns.

The Role of Hormones in Your Health

Nearly every preceding chapter of this book offers some information about hormones—their role in your body and the impact of changing hormone levels on your health. But as you move into the decision about hormone therapy, it's important that you remember a few of the more important facts about hormones. For example, though your body produces a number of hormones, three hormones play leading roles in your reproductive cycle: estrogen, progesterone, and androgens. All three of these hormones can be used in hormone therapy and therefore may continue to play a role in your health from puberty through your mature years.

Because hormones are such an important and widely used tool for controlling menopausal symptoms, including hot flashes, night sweats, mood swings, vaginal atrophy, and later, bone loss and deteriorating vision, they are the subject of constant, ongoing medical research.

The Women's Health Initiative (WHI) Study

In 1991 the National Institutes of Health began a fifteen-year study of over 150,000 women, age fifty to seventy-nine, that was designed to examine a number of factors as they relate to the prevention of heart disease, cancer, and osteoporosis. One subsection of this enormous study was a clinical trial study involving 68,000 postmenopausal women. These women could participate in any or all three of three preventive approaches: hormone therapy, dietary modifications, and/or calcium and vitamin D supplementation.

 Fact

> There are many terms to refer to hormone therapy. "HRT" refers to Hormone Replacement Therapy. A variation of that, "ERT" stands for Estrogen Replacement Therapy. Since some scientists maintain that they are not "replacing" but rather "creating" a hormonal environment, the terms "MHT," for menopausal hormone therapy, and "HT," for hormone therapy are becoming more common. "ET" usually refers to Estrogen Therapy, without other hormones, and "EPT" to Estrogen combined with Progestin Therapy.

The hormone therapy study was randomly divided between placebo groups and estrogen, or estrogen and progestin, therapies. Women taking either placebo or hormone regimens were studied to determine their risk for cardiovascular disease and cancer. During the first five years of the study, the percentage of woman between the ages of fifty and seventy-four using MHT went from 33 percent to 42 percent. It was conventional wisdom at that time that using estrogen would delay heart disease, osteoporosis, and aging in general.

In 2002, study findings were beginning to show that not only was hormone therapy *not* protective against heart disease and stroke, but that women on hormones actually had an *increased* risk of those conditions. The study was stopped, and women were advised not to go on hormone therapy to prevent heart disease and/or stroke. Women and their physicians were left confused and wondering how to deal with this information. Thousands of women were taken off estrogen and other hormone combinations, and prescriptions for hormone therapy dropped 38 percent in the first year following publication of the results.

Since then, scientists have analyzed the data to determine more clearly what the risks are and in what cases hormone therapy may be advisable for women. Recent evidence suggests that women are returning slowly to use of MHT, but for shorter periods of time, and at lower doses. These benefits and risks will be described later, but for the latest developments and findings from the WHI study, go to *www.nih.gov/PHTindex.htm*.

Estrogen and Its Use in MHT

Estrogen is a growth hormone that stimulates the development of adult sex organs during puberty. Estrogen helps retain calcium in bones, a function that keeps bones strong and whole during childbearing years. It also regulates the balance of cholesterol in the bloodstream and helps lower your body's total cholesterol level (see Menopause and Heart Disease in Chapter 14). Estrogen aids other body functions, such as regulating blood sugar levels and emotional balance. It helps keep skin supple and elastic through its nonstop job of replacing dead cells and maintaining proper collagen structure (the basic structural component of skin and supporting structures). Similarly, it promotes healthy, well-nourished vaginal tissue to help maintain flexible, moist, and elastic vaginal walls.

 Alert

If you have your uterus, your health care professional won't prescribe unopposed estrogen for treatment of menopausal symptoms. Be aware, however, that if you self-medicate with plant estrogens (phytoestrogens) from soy foods or supplements, you may be giving your body unopposed estrogens. Talk to your health care provider about any and all supplements and vitamins you take on a regular basis.

The amount of hormones your ovaries are able to secrete gradually diminishes in your late forties, so your body produces lower amounts of estrogen and other hormones. In the early stages of perimenopause, the pituitary gland in the brain produces its own hormones to try to stimulate the ovaries to produce more estrogen, and it works, for a while. The ovaries occasionally are able to develop an egg that produces enough estrogen to trigger a menstrual period. However, in this transition phase a woman may experience widely fluctuating levels of estrogen for a number of years, until the ovaries shut down completely. The body continues to produce small amounts of estrogen, but only at about 25 percent or less of its premenopause rate—levels too small to support the hormone's age-defying functions in the body.

Estrogen is used in MHT to:

- Diminish hot flashes
- Keep the vaginal walls supple, moist, and well nourished
- Maintain or even increase bone density
- Help alleviate urinary tract problems and diminish stress and urge incontinence
- Lower the risk of age-related macular degeneration of the eye and glaucoma (when used with progestin)
- Lower the risk of rheumatoid arthritis and improve the motor symptoms of Parkinson's disease

Estrogen's powerful benefits have resulted in its use for perimenopausal symptoms for more than fifty years. In the 1950s and 1960s, many doctors prescribed unopposed estrogen replacement—meaning that the woman received estrogen alone—without the balancing effects of the hormone progesterone, even if she had an intact uterus. But later studies revealed that estrogen given alone could result in the development of endometrial cancer, so MHT today almost always involves some combination of estrogen, progesterone, and in some cases, androgens such as testosterone. If a woman has had a hysterectomy, she doesn't need to worry about endometrial cancer, so her hormone prescription may be estrogen alone, known as ET, estrogen therapy.

Estrogen Therapy

Estrogens offer many health benefits, but these powerful hormones can have some negative effects. Estrogen can contribute to the occurrence of blood clots in the deep veins of the legs or the lungs of women who have a history of these problems.

Fact

> It was thought that estrogen might prevent the onset of Alzheimer's disease or other types of dementia, but the Women's Health Initiative (WHI) study did not show that at all. In fact, there was some indication that women taking estrogen might develop these conditions sooner. As with other findings in this study, the results will be refined to determine which women are at greatest risk. In the meantime, MHT is not recommended for prevention of dementia and memory loss.

As you progress through perimenopause, your body's hormonal changes take place over a period of months or years, giving your system time to adjust to gradually declining hormone levels. If you go through an induced menopause—for example, following the surgical removal of the ovaries—your menopause will be immediate and probably dramatic in its physical impact. In those cases, your doctor or health care provider is likely to recommend some form of estrogen therapy to help your body through the transition.

Progesterone and Its Use in MHT

Progesterone is an important hormone, though its benefits and impact may seem less dramatic than those of estrogen. Normally, your ovaries produce progesterone in the process of ovulation, so most women in their reproductive years that report having regular menstrual cycles would be expected to have normal progesterone levels. Progesterone stabilizes the growth of your uterine lining (endometrium) thereby limiting the quantity of your menstrual blood flow. In your childbearing years, progesterone also promotes the development of nutrients in the uterus, breasts, and fallopian tubes to prepare your body for supporting a pregnancy.

E. Essential

> One of the promising results from the WHI study was the impact of MHT on hip fractures and colorectal cancers. Both were reduced in women taking hormone therapy, so if you are at increased risk of osteoporosis or have a strong family history of colorectal cancer, discuss this with your health care provider when deciding whether MHT is for you.

Your progesterone levels drop dramatically when you stop ovulating. Because progesterone's most important effect in your body is its estrogen-balancing capabilities, most MHT prescriptions for women who still have a uterus include some type of progestin, a pharmaceutical form of the naturally occurring hormone progesterone.

In spite of its critical importance for balancing the effects of estrogen, progestin has its drawbacks. Some women experience breast tenderness and water retention when taking progestin with estrogen in an MHT regimen. Other women find that some forms of progestin aggravate mood swings. And many forms of progestin can diminish the heart-healthy effects of estrogen, which is why doctors usually don't include progestin therapy in MHT if a woman has had a hysterectomy.

For these reasons, doctors and health care providers monitor hormone therapy patients carefully to determine which progestin type and delivery technique works best for each individual. If you have a medical history of high cholesterol, discuss this history with your doctor before deciding on an MHT prescription.

A number of different types of progestins are available, and it can be taken continuously, cyclically (twelve to fourteen days of every month), or in a pulsed regimen of three days on and three days off. Progestins given in a cyclic fashion usually produce a predictable menstrual period; progestins given in the same dose on a daily basis are designed to make most women period-free after one year of therapy or sooner.

Androgens in MHT

Androgens are male hormones that are normally produced in small quantities by the ovaries and adrenal glands, with the greatest quantities occurring at the midpoint of a woman's cycle. Androgens contribute to bone density (though not as dramatically as do estrogens), and some studies show that they might promote a healthy libido by fostering a desire for sex. Androgen production also drops dramatically when ovarian function decreases around the time of perimenopause. The decrease is even more dramatic if a woman undergoes a surgical menopause. If women have severe menopausal or perimenopausal symptoms, such as intermittent hot flashes or a greatly reduced sex drive, despite a trial of traditional MHT, their health care providers may recommend an MHT regimen that includes androgens.

The use of androgens to combat menopausal symptoms is relatively new, unlike estrogen, which has been used and studied since the mid-1950s. Some studies have shown that androgen in combination with estrogen not only slows bone loss but also may help promote the growth of new bone tissue. Some experts believe androgens help alleviate other menopausal symptoms such as hot flashes and vaginal dryness. Androgens carry some risks, of course; some studies suggest that androgen can have a negative effect on blood cholesterol levels, and a few patients who take androgens can experience unwanted side effects such as the growth of excess body hair (especially on the face), acne, or oiliness of the skin. In general, androgens are added to an MHT regimen only if libido or hot flashes are not improved on standard MHT dosages.

 Fact

More than half of the women who experience irregular spotting or bleeding after beginning an MHT regimen that includes progestin stop bleeding completely after six months; 80 percent stop bleeding within a year. Continued bleeding (after one year) may indicate a problem with the lining of the uterus, rather than a reaction to MHT.

The Facts about MHT

Perimenopausal and postmenopausal women have a variety of alternatives for protecting their health and treating menopausal symptoms. The most common and studied of these is hormone therapy. Both women and their providers have more reservations about beginning hormone therapy, and in truth, MHT isn't for everyone. Your personal risk profile may make you a poor candidate for hormone therapy. Or you may be a person who chooses "natural" or "alternative" ways to maintain your health and alleviate menopausal symptoms. Whatever choices you make should be based on fact—not on unnecessary fears or unfounded beliefs about the safety or positive impact of this treatment option.

Who Uses MHT?

Menopause hormone therapy is used by fewer than half of all menopausal women in the United States. The reasons for using—or not using—MHT vary from individual to individual, but many women who aren't on MHT are still deciding whether it is a good option for them. Whatever technique you use to minimize postmenopausal bone loss, heart disease, muscle and other tissue degradation, memory function loss, and other effects of diminished hormones, it's best to decide before the hormone levels get extremely low. Here's what we know about the women who choose MHT and why they choose it:

- Most surveys indicate that the main reason women between the ages of fifty and fifty-five choose to begin MHT is for the relief of hot flashes and other vasomotor symptoms. Women who begin MHT at age sixty-five and older are more likely to be concerned with preventing or postponing the onset of osteoporosis.
- About 35 percent of perimenopausal women turn to MHT for the relief of night sweats and vaginal dryness—in addition to hot flashes.
- A 1997 survey reported in the Journal of Women's Health discovered that nearly 50 percent of those who were currently using MHT had undergone a hysterectomy. In that study, over 35 percent of current MHT users and over 40 percent of past users

turned to MHT as a result of surgically induced menopause. Understandably, women who no longer have a uterus have little concern over irregular vaginal bleeding.

The Benefits of MHT

MHT offers women a number of sound, solid health benefits—both in the relief of symptoms and in the prevention of some serious health threats that result from the body's loss of hormones.

MHT has proven its benefit in maintaining bone health and preventing osteoporosis. Most studies show that women who use estrogen and progestin MHT compounds reduce their risk of hip fracture by 11 percent for each year of MHT treatments. Here are just some of the other benefits of hormone replacement therapy:

- MHT is the most time-proven method for reducing hot flashes, vaginal dryness, and other uncomfortable menopausal symptoms.
- Estrogen may be effective in protecting the eyes from macular degeneration—the leading cause of blindness in those age sixty-five and older. Macular degeneration is the most common cause of failures for the eye examination required in the driver's license recertification process. A lack of the ability to drive a car is one of the most common causes of loss of independence and feelings of isolation and depression among the elderly.
- Estrogen reduces the risk of contracting colorectal cancer by as much as a third in most studies.

 Fact

Macular degeneration often takes the form of a clouding of the eye's lens. Age-related macular degeneration (AMD) causes the retina to deteriorate, and it's usually noticeable first as a clouding of the central area of vision (the peripheral vision can remain intact). AMD is the leading cause of night blindness in the United States. Many doctors recommend MHT to prevent or delay AMD.

Your personal risk profile and family history can help you and your health care provider assess the benefits of MHT for you.

The Risks of MHT

It is obvious that hormone therapy can be advantageous for many women during and after the menopausal years, but it is just as obvious that the risks need to be weighed against those possible benefits. New studies are always refining our understanding of these risks.

Breast Cancer

When the WHI study results were announced in 2002, millions of women stopped taking MHT. This created a unique opportunity to see the resulting effect on breast cancer rates. In 2006, the rates were reported to have dropped 7 percent in the year 2003—one year after women stopped taking hormones. Although this doesn't prove a link between MHT and breast cancer, it strongly suggests it. The type of cancers most affected were the estrogen-sensitive cancers, further suggesting this link. Although the overall risk of breast cancer is still small, most health care professionals advise women who have a personal history of breast cancer against using MHT for at least the first five years following their diagnoses. Regardless of their use of MHT or family history, all menopausal women should get regular mammograms, conduct monthly self-breast exams, and visit their physician annually.

Endometrial Cancer

If you still have your uterus, you shouldn't take unopposed estrogen (estrogen without progesterone) for the sole purpose of relief of menopausal symptoms, because unopposed estrogen can increase your risk of developing endometrial cancer. MHT programs that balance estrogen with progestin decrease this risk, however, and may in fact help reduce the risk of endometrial cancer even further compared to women who take no hormone supplements. If you have been treated successfully for early (stages I through III) endometrial cancer, with a total hysterectomy, your doctor may recommend an ET regimen for you after a certain disease-free interval, usually three to five years.

Blood Clots

If you have ever developed blood clots in the deep veins of your legs or in your lungs or eyes, you may be susceptible to redeveloping them if you use MHT. High levels of estrogen can contribute to this condition, so your health care professional will want to test your current blood hormone levels and review your history to see if you are a good candidate for MHT. Your doctor can order special blood tests that check for clotting difficulties if your family or personal medical history raises any question about an inherited susceptibility.

 Fact

Irregular bleeding or spotting is the most common side effect complaint of women on MHT, while others report breast tenderness and water retention. And, while some women say MHT contributes to migraines, others say it actually helps ameliorate migraine problems they've experienced for years.

Liver Disease

If you have active liver disease or if your liver's functions have become seriously impaired through illness or injury, you aren't a good candidate for MHT. If your liver isn't functioning properly, your body won't be able to metabolize the estrogen component of MHT.

MHT Options

Because MHT is such a widely used and studied method of treatment, a number of different MHT compounds and delivery methods have developed over the years. You and your doctor can determine the form that's best for you, but here are some of the most popular options:

- Pills can offer estrogen or estrogen/progestin combinations that are taken continuously, cyclically, or in pulse patterns of, for example, three days on then three days off.

Alert

Not all hormone creams and gels are approved by the Food and Drug Administration (FDA). Be sure to consult your physician regarding proper dosage, possible side effects, and application of these creams.

- Patches can deliver a steady dose of estrogen or estrogen/ progestin combinations every day of the month. You change patches every three to seven days, and you can wear them when swimming or showering.
- Flexible vaginal rings deliver estrogen in steady doses to women who suffer from vaginal dryness. Some forms are available that make estrogen replacement safe even for breast cancer patients, because the estrogen works locally (in the vagina), and is not absorbed into the bloodstream (which could increase the potential for the recurrence of the cancer).
- Creams and gels provide topical estrogen or progesterone doses to women who suffer from vaginal dryness. Both creams and gels are applied directly inside the vagina; some women rub vaginal progesterone gels and creams directly on the skin. Again, your health care provider can advise you on the proper dose and delivery mechanism for these (and all) forms of MHT.

Low-Dose MHT

The Food and Drug Administration (FDA) has approved new formulations of estrogen/progestin that are much lower than combinations used prior to the WHI study. These formulations seem to offer good protection from osteoporosis, when women also take vitamin D and calcium. It is unclear yet whether these lower doses have the same risks as higher doses for cardiovascular disease and other conditions.

Bioidentical Hormones

Bioidentical hormones have been highlighted in the popular media. With celebrities touting them as the "safe" alternatives to conventional conjugated hormones, and declaring them a virtual fountain of youth, many women are curious about them. Also called "natural hormones," bioidentical hormones are formulated to be exactly the same chemical as that produced naturally by the ovaries. The ovaries produce three types of estrogen: estradiol, estrone, and estriol. These formulations can be duplicated from plant sources, creating a chemical twin to what your body produces. Estradiol is available in FDA-approved forms, such as tablets, skin patches, and vaginal forms. Estriol and estrone are available from compounding pharmacies. Bioidentical progesterone is also available as tablets and vaginal gel, and from compounding pharmacies.

 Fact

The FDA recommends a balanced approach to prescribing either traditional MHT or the newer "low-dose" MHT formulations. The bottom line for you and your health care provider is this: If you are going to try MHT, use the lowest effective dose for the shortest period of time.

Proponents of bioidenticals point out that compounding pharmacies can create individual formulations that will meet each woman's particular hormone needs according to her symptoms and risks. Critics of bioidenticals suggest that compounding pharmacies produce an uneven product that can vary from batch to batch, and that some of the inactive ingredients will differ and affect the action of the hormone. The FDA-approved versions can offer a more proven safety record but are not as individualized.

The most controversial assumption about bioidentical hormones is that they are safer than their synthetic counterparts are. This remains to be seen, since they have not yet been studied side by side with the synthetic versions, and therefore may have all the same risks as those discovered in the WHI study.

Essential

When trying to assess how risky bioidentical hormones are as compared to synthetic hormones, information is very sparse. The WHI
study did not include bioidentical formulations, so it is hard to say
whether they would have shown the same risk factors as hormones
used in the study.

Designer Estrogens

In the past several years, a number of artificial estrogens have been
developed to provide some of the benefits of estrogen replacement
therapy while avoiding some of the risks for women who aren't good
candidates for MHT. In other words, the artificial estrogens act like
estrogens with some of the body's tissues, but they don't act like estrogens with others. These so-called "designer estrogens" are more cor-
rectly referred to as selective estrogen receptor modulators or SERMs.
Some health care providers prescribe SERMs to combat bone loss in
postmenopausal patients who can't or choose not to use MHT but who
are at risk of developing osteoporosis. Following are the most common
SERMs in use today:

- Tamoxifen (sold under the brand name Nolvadex) has been in
  use for some years to help reduce the potential for recurrence of
  estrogen-dependent breast cancer in women with a history of that
  disease. Ongoing study and scrutiny of Tamoxifen indicate that it
  isn't an "ideal answer" for postmenopausal women. Some studies
  have linked it to an increased risk of endometrial polyps, blood
  clots, and possibly precancerous endometrial hyperplasia.
- Raloxifene was approved by the FDA in 1997 for use in the prevention of osteoporosis, and was marketed in 1998 under the
  brand name Evista. Though still under study, raloxifene has
  been found to maintain a certain amount of bone density in
  some patients, without increasing the risk of breast or uterine

cancer. Because it doesn't appear to have any adverse effects on the endometrium, women who still have their uterus don't need to take progestin or progesterone when on raloxifene. However, some studies show that raloxifene is only about half as effective as estrogen at increasing bone density. Raloxifene's effect on cholesterol is still unknown; though it appears to reduce LDL cholesterol, it hasn't been shown to increase "good" HDL cholesterol the way estrogen does. The risk of blood clots with raloxifene seems to be similar to that of estrogen, and raloxifene has shown no beneficial effect in reducing hot flashes. It actually increases hot flashes in some patients.

SERMs show great promise for postmenopausal treatment without the risks of traditional hormones. They are typically used for treatment of bone loss, and more recently, for vaginal atrophy. New versions of this category of drug are being developed, and side effects are being studied to see whether they are a good substitute for hormones in women who have those symptoms.

 ## Fact

Lasofoxifene, one of the newer SERMs, was shown, at a 2005 meeting of the North American Menopause Society (NAMS), to relieve the symptoms of vaginal atrophy, and is the first SERM to definitively improve this menopausal symptom.

Weighing Risks and Benefits

So how do you decide whether to use MHT or what form of MHT is best for you? You've probably guessed the answer to this one—talk with your doctor or health care professional. Educating yourself about the risks and benefits of MHT is a good first step, but you can always benefit from a professional's firsthand experience and advice when making this decision. When you meet with your health care professional, ask about the following tests and risks factors:

- Talk to your doctor about your personal and family history of osteoporosis, heart disease, breast cancer, blood clots, colon cancer, and liver disease.
- Ask about a bone density test to determine the current state of your bone health.
- Request a fasting blood test called a lipid profile to find out your levels of total cholesterol, HDL, LDL, and triglycerides to determine your cardiac disease risk.
- Ask about the usefulness of blood tests to determine your current blood hormone levels, or how close you are to menopause.
- Keep your menstrual journal or menstrual symptom diary (see Appendix B: Keeping a Menopause Journal) and take it with you to discuss the symptoms you've been having and their severity, so you know what kind of symptom relief you need most.
- Ask your doctor or health care professional about alternatives to MHT, their benefits, and their drawbacks.

Part of a Healthy Menopause Plan

Hormone therapy offers a number of benefits for women in perimenopause, menopause, and postmenopause. But lifestyle and behavioral changes are an important part of a complete plan for a healthy life—before, during, and after the onset of menopause. No pill, patch, or cream will keep you healthy if you live an unhealthy lifestyle. As you grow older, your health maintenance becomes more critical—and more demanding.

Essential

Remember to follow your MHT program exactly as prescribed. Many people forget their schedule and miss doses. Use whatever reminder mechanism works for you—a weekly pill container, a marked calendar, notes on your mirror, or other device. If you can't find a reminder that works, ask your health care professional for advice. But don't miss doses!

NoReplacement for a Healthy Lifestyle

Even if you adopt a full program of MHT—or use any MHT alternative—you need to follow the guidelines listed below to maintain your good health:

- Eat a healthy diet that's high in vegetables, fruits, and whole grains, and low in saturated fat and red meat. Maintaining strong muscles, healthy bones, and good heart health requires a good diet.
- Get plenty of exercise. Weight-bearing exercise, such as walking or weightlifting, improves the health of your heart, develops muscle mass, reduces body fat, and builds strong bones. The best MHT program in the world won't protect your health if you turn into a couch potato.
- Get plenty of sleep. Sleep deprivation contributes to anxiety, depression, and fatigue—the most troublesome symptoms of hormone depletion.
- Stop smoking. Smoking not only harms your health but also increases your risk for certain types of cancers that are more common in menopause. Smoking and estrogen are a bad combination; do yourself and everyone who loves you a favor, and kick the habit.
- Get regular medical checkups. Your doctor will recommend annual examinations to monitor the progress of your MHT program. During the exam, your health care provider will check your breasts for lumps; do a pelvic exam to determine the health of your uterus, cervix, vagina, and ovaries; and check your blood pressure. Preventive care is an important part of your MHT program. Ask about screening for colon cancer as well.

You Are One of a Kind

As with all elements of menopause, the decision about MHT is unique to you and your personal goals and risk factors. It does carry risks, as outlined earlier. But it is also very effective for treating some of the debilitating symptoms of hormone loss. A cautious approach of using the lowest doses for only the time necessary to treat your symptoms seems to be the best approach. Research continues, so stay tuned!

CHAPTER 12

Alternatives to MHT

HORMONE THERAPY ISN'T THE ANSWER for every woman's menopausal symptom relief. Many women choose not to use traditional MHT, and others aren't suitable candidates for MHT because of a personal or family medical history. If you are among these women—or are simply interested in learning more about nonhormonal treatment options—this chapter provides some information about alternatives.

Why Some Women Choose MHT Alternatives

Hormone therapy is only one way to deal with menopausal symptoms. As the risks and benefits of hormone therapy are discovered, women want to understand all the alternatives for making this transition a comfortable and healthy one.

Women Want Choices

Medical complications aren't the only issue that might send a woman in search of an alternative to MHT. Women have many reasons for choosing alternatives to hormones, including the following:

- **Troublesome side effects of MHT.** Many women who begin MHT decide for themselves to discontinue its use, citing progestin-related side effects including vaginal bleeding, breast tenderness, bloating, depression, and irritability.
- **Fear of an increased risk of cancer.** Research seems to indicate that MHT can increase the risk of estrogen-sensitive breast cancers. If a woman has a personal or family history of breast cancer, she may want to avoid even the small chance of increasing her risk.

- **Objection to the "medicalization" of a natural process.** Many women see menopause, like puberty, to be a normal, anticipated stage of physical development, and therefore want to approach it with as little medical intervention as possible. The North American Menopause Society (NAMS) found that nearly half of American women surveyed considered menopause a natural process that doesn't require medical management. The National Institutes of Health (NIH) supports dissemination of information "that emphasizes menopause as a normal, healthy phase of women's lives and promotes it demedicalization."

Each individual must educate herself about all treatment options and then work closely with a trusted health care professional to make this highly personal choice. Take advantage of the benefits of scientific advancements and research that are available for improving the quality of your life.

Other reasons may be factors in discouraging women from using MHT. Many women haven't the funds for ongoing medical therapy and are uninsured or underinsured, and therefore can't afford it. These women face multiple challenges in finding affordable alternatives to MHT, since many alternative treatments are also costly, and are even less likely to be covered by insurance. Some women may choose to avoid any kind of medical treatment as a result of religious or philosophical beliefs. For these women, nonmedical alternatives to MHT offer acceptable options for maintaining physical and emotional health during the transition through menopause.

 Alert

Alternative therapies can be expensive. One survey found that the average vitamin/mineral/nutritional menopause symptom treatment costs about $2.00 per tablet—essentially the same as the cost of the usual dose of MHT.

Remember the Medical Impacts of Menopause

If you choose not to take MHT for either medical or personal reasons, you need to adopt other means of protecting your bones, brain, skin, and heart as you age. Any treatment option you choose must be part of a balanced, lifelong program of healthy living. Diet, exercise, regular medical checkups, and an active, engaged lifestyle are critical to preserving your ongoing health—through menopause and beyond.

Essential

Don't look to any one source—especially popular consumer magazines or blogs on the Internet—for information about menopause. Check the Resources section (Appendix C) for other sources of sound information. Talk to your health care provider and other health care professionals to get second—even third—opinions.

Nonhormonal Medications

Many women use nonhormonal prescription medications to combat the initial symptoms of menopause, including hot flashes, insomnia, sexual dysfunction, depression, mood swings, and fatigue. Medical treatments and preventatives for some physical conditions such as cholesterol imbalances, high blood pressure, bone loss, and vaginal dryness also are available. This section offers a brief overview of some of the most widely prescribed and effective nonhormonal prescription medications in use for the treatment of menopause symptoms. Check with your health care provider about what he or she might be willing to prescribe for you.

For Hot Flashes and Night Sweats

As discussed in Chapter 5, even though MHT is still considered the gold standard for treatment of hot flashes and vasomotor symptoms, there are several nonhormonal remedies for hot flashes. For women avoiding hormones, prescription drugs such as clonidine, some antidepressants, and gabapentin can offer significant relief from hot flashes. Herbal remedies are mentioned later in this chapter.

 Fact

> Many women who have a personal history of breast cancer turn to nonhormonal prescription medications for the control of hot flashes and night sweats. Research continues to refine the medical world's knowledge of these drugs and their impact on vasomotor symptoms.

For Blood Pressure and Cholesterol Management

Although estrogen has been shown to be an effective tool for normalizing cholesterol levels in women as they pass through menopause, it is not a good treatment for high cholesterol.

Diet and exercise are your two most effective means for controlling cholesterol levels and blood pressure. But many medications are currently available to treat both conditions:

- The so-called "statins" (Simvastatin, Pravastatin, and Lovastatin) are very effective in lowering cholesterol levels and preventing deaths due to heart disease. These drugs can interact with some other medications, and they aren't recommended for people with active liver disease.
- Diuretics flush water and sodium from the body and can be effective for reducing blood pressure. They reduce the level of fluid in your bloodstream and help remove sodium from your circulation, so they may help open up and boost the capacity of your arteries, which lowers the blood pressure against your arterial walls.
- Beta-blockers, including lopranolol and metoprolol, block some of the nerve impulses to the heart, making the heartbeat slower and the heart's workload decrease.

- ACE inhibitors are also effective in controlling high blood pressure, and they seem to work by inhibiting the formation of a substance that causes blood vessels to constrict.
- Calcium channel blockers slow the movement of calcium into the blood vessels and heart cells, relaxing the vessels and increasing the amount of blood to the heart. They are often prescribed to reduce blood pressure, but they also slow the heart rate and can make you drowsy until you get used to them.

High blood pressure medications have a range of possible side effects, and most doctors recommend lifestyle changes as a first line of defense against this disease.

Essential

If you have access to the Internet, you can turn to the National Institutes of Health's National Medical Library for authoritative information about most drugs prescribed today. Use the Library's topic list, drug information, and dictionaries to find out how any drug works, how it's prescribed, and its potential side effects and interactions. Find the library at *www.nlm.nih.gov* (click on "MEDLINEplus").

For Managing Bone Loss

Though estrogen is the undisputed queen of bone maintenance, medical science has made a number of strides in finding alternative drugs that slow the bone loss associated with menopause. Weight-bearing exercise and a diet rich in calcium and vitamin D are important components of any plan to maintain good bone health. For details on medications used to fight osteoporosis, see Chapter 15.

For Combating Insomnia, Depression, and Anxiety

Though thousands of people in the United States suffer from sleep disorders, insomnia becomes a true enemy of women as they approach menopause. Hormonal fluctuations lead to night sweats and mild panic attacks that can blast a woman out of a sound sleep at 3 A.M. and keep her awake for hours.

 Fact

> The National Sleep Foundation (NSF) recommends that any type of sleep-aiding medication be used only in conjunction with lifestyle changes, including diet restrictions, exercise, a regular sleep schedule, and a managed sleep environment. Even then, the NSF recommends that use of the sleep aids be short term or intermittent.

Lifestyle changes are essential to guarding your sleep and leading a calm, rested, and energetic life. Exercise, stress-management techniques, and a diet low in caffeine and alcohol all are important components of any plan to maintain deep, restful sleep and emotional health. Though doctors sometimes recommend MHT for the relief of insomnia, depression, and anxiety, a number of medications are also available to help menopausal women combat these debilitating conditions.

Insomnia treatment is detailed in Chapter 7, so consult that chapter for details on the use of several medications.

Treatment of depression may be achieved with the same lifestyle choices mentioned previously, including healthy diet, regular exercise, and daily sunlight. Additionally, there are many medication choices such as selective serotonin reuptake inhibitor (SSRI) antidepressants (see Chapter 8 for more detail on treatment of depression). Your health care provider may refer you to someone familiar with medication choices if depression is a major symptom during menopause.

Anxiety can be treated with anti-anxiety drugs such as buspirone and alprazolam. These medications, called anxiolytics, also can treat the symptoms of premenstrual dysphoric disorder (PMDD) that many perimenopausal women experience as they move closer to menopause.

These drugs can have a slightly sedative effect, so many health care professionals prescribe them only for short periods of time.

Prescription medications can offer true relief from many of the symptoms and physical conditions that result from perimenopause and menopause. But they aren't your only—and many times not even the best—answer. Some combination of prescription medications and/or hormone therapy may help temporarily treat many menopausal symptoms, but lifestyle choices are always the best tools for maintaining your health and emotional well-being. The following sections discuss supplemental vitamins and nutrients and a range of therapeutic programs that can also help keep you strong, fit, and healthy through menopause.

 Alert

If you have sleep apnea or have to operate heavy machinery soon after awakening, your doctor is unlikely to recommend hypnotics as treatment for insomnia. Hypnotics can actually make breathing even more difficult for those with sleep apnea, and some hypnotics can continue having an impact on brain functions long enough to impair your abilities shortly after awakening.

Choosing Natural Alternatives Wisely

You've probably noticed the ever-growing selection of herbal compounds and other botanical treatments available for the management of menopausal symptoms. Frequent articles in magazines and newspapers and on the Web discuss the latest vitamin or herbal alternatives, and the scientific community continues to test and release results on the effectiveness of these compounds for the treatment of specific physical or emotional disorders. Because botanical extracts and nutritional supplements aren't subject to Food and Drug Administration (FDA) approval, each consumer is responsible for making the wisest, most informed choice when buying these products.

You Be the Judge

The need for information for women seeking a natural alternative to MHT for the relief of menopausal symptoms is especially critical; the alternatives must offer relief from a range of symptoms while at the same time supplementing the body's supply of important vitamins and minerals.

Consider the following important points when you're assessing the value of choosing herbs and/or nutritional supplements for the treatment of menopausal symptoms:

1. **Are you looking for symptom relief or health maintenance?** Many herbal alternatives are effective for relieving a single symptom or for supplementing a specific nutritional need. The wider the range of relief you are seeking, the more pills, capsules, powders, and teas you may need to consume. And you will need your health care professional to assess the safety of that combination.

2. **Have you already adopted the healthy lifestyle changes recommended for women at your stage of life?** A proper diet, regular exercise, and good stress-management skills are as essential for those using alternative treatments for menopausal symptoms as they are for women using MHT. No botanical compound, vitamin collection, or nutritional supplement will replace these very basic necessities for maintaining your health through menopause.

3. **Have you talked with others who are using the treatment alternative you're considering, and have you discussed it with your health care provider?** Making a decision to use these alternatives requires that you educate yourself on all of the possible benefits and drawbacks of your choice. Your choice of botanical and nutritional supplements that are powerful enough to treat the symptoms and diminish the physical degradation of bone, muscle, and brain tissue accompanying menopause could actually be dangerous, and requires careful consideration.

L., Essential

Plant substances aren't inherently safer or more benign than laboratory produced chemicals, and are not subject to FDA approval. Plant
extracts can be very powerful and can interact with prescription or
nonprescription drugs to cause dangerous side effects. Don't take
any substance without fully understanding its effects, and ask your
health care provider if it's safe for you.

Explore Your Options

The range of botanical substances, nutritional supplements, and
nutraceuticals available for perimenopausal and menopausal women is
vast. Appendix C contains a number of authoritative references for more
information on this topic. The following sections list some of the most
popular—and promising—herbs, nutritional supplements, and plant
extracts in use today for management of menopausal symptoms.

Herbs and Other Supplements

Dietary supplements are defined by the Dietary Supplement Health and
Education Act (DSHEA) of 1994 as "products that contains substances
like vitamins, minerals, foods, botanicals, amino acids and which are
intended to supplement the usual intake of these substances." Herbal
remedies are also known as botanicals, and are a subset of the larger
group of dietary and nutritional supplements.

Women have been using herbs to combat the symptoms of menopause for centuries—in fact, only in the past century have any other
options been available. As pharmaceutical science has evolved over the
past hundred years, so has our understanding of the benefits of supplementing a healthy diet with vitamin and mineral compounds. Today,
nearly every woman takes some form of vitamin, herb, or nutritional
supplement at some time—if not throughout her life. Most health care
experts recommend that women supplement a healthy diet with certain
vitamins and minerals as they approach menopause.

Many women turn to botanical compounds, plant and herb extracts, and nutritional supplements to alleviate the symptoms of perimenopause and to offset the physical changes the body can experience because of lowered estrogen and the natural aging process.

 Fact

Complementary and alternative remedies for menopausal and age-related symptoms must be weighed carefully against pharmaceutical choices. When deciding on a plan to maintain your long-term health during and after menopause, get the authoritative information and advice you need to make an intelligent decision.

Black Cohosh

Black cohosh is perhaps one of the most popular herbal remedies used for the management of menopausal symptoms. Native American women have used its roots for centuries for relief of a number of symptoms associated with menstruation and menopause. Long-term studies through the National Institutes of Health (NIH) have shown it to be only as effective as placebo in treating menopausal symptoms.

In previous studies, black cohosh was found to lower luteinizing hormone (LH) levels by binding to certain estrogen receptors. Double-blind tests conducted on Remifem, an over-the-counter supplement that contains black cohosh, found that some participants felt some relief from symptoms including hot flashes, depression-like symptoms, and occasional sleeplessness. It has a good safety record so far and is still being studied for its potential in treating menopausal symptoms.

It's not clear whether black cohosh is safe for women with breast cancer and other estrogen-sensitive cancers. Side effects of black cohosh include nausea, vomiting, dizziness, and at least one reported case of nocturnal seizures, and it should not be used during pregnancy as it may cause miscarriage or premature birth. In menopause or peri-menopause, its use is not recommended for more than six months.

Gingko Biloba

Many women turn to gingko biloba supplements, extracted from the leaf of the gingko biloba tree, as treatment for the mental fogginess that seems to descend upon them as menopause approaches. Gingko biloba has been studied in placebo-controlled tests and shown to work better than a placebo at aiding memory and concentration. Gingko has been shown to improve circulation and may, therefore, aid the supply of nourishment to the brain through the circulatory system. Results of studies have been mixed. The National Institute on Aging has studied the use of this extract in the treatment of Alzheimer's disease, but did not see significant effectiveness. The National Institutes of Health (NIH), through its National Center for Complimentary and Alternative Medicine (NCCAM), is conducting a longer-term study of 3,000 volunteers to determine whether gingko biloba can reduce or delay the onset of dementia, and what effect it has on cardiovascular disease. Typical dosages of gingko are forty to eighty milligrams (taken in capsule form) three times daily. Most sources indicate that you need to take this dosage for up to twelve weeks in order to feel the effect. Talk to your health care provider for the latest information about dosage and appropriateness for your symptoms.

Kava

Also known as *kawa,* or *kava kava,* this member of the pepper family is used for anxiety and insomnia. Sometimes called "the intoxicating pepper," the root of the plant has been shown to have its greatest usefulness as an anti-anxiety agent, and it has not been proven effective in reducing hot flashes. Kava is addictive and can cause extreme drowsiness if you use it while drinking alcohol or taking antihistamines. The FDA has issued a warning that it may be associated with liver damage, linking it to at least twenty-five cases worldwide. So while the danger of liver problems is low, it does seem to exist with this botanical.

Finding Out about Other Herbs and Supplements

This chapter has explored only the most commonly used compounds and nutritional supplements available for the treatment of menopausal symptoms. Others include:

- Chasteberry (in Latin *vitus agnus castus*) is said to balance hormonal fluctuations. Thought to act on the pituitary, it is used to relieve hot flashes, vaginal dryness, and depression. It is used for many uterine conditions and is also a libido balancer and lactation stimulant. It interacts with hormones and some other medications, so you should talk to your medical provider before using it.

- Dong quai, believed by some to treat hot flashes, was found ineffective in recent studies and may increase the flow of menstrual blood. Other side effects include photosensitivity and photodermatitis (sun rash), and it may cause cancer or mutations or increase the effects of the drug warfarin (Coumadin—a frequently prescribed blood thinner) and antiplatelet agents.

- SAMe (S-Adenosylmethionine) shows good evidence that it can repair damaged cartilage for better joint health. It is also being studied for its use as an antidepressant, and while promising the results are not yet definitive. SAMe does seem to have a good safety record. However, it can interact with some medications for Parkinson's disease and with other antidepressants.

- Ginseng root is considered by many to aid well-being, mood, and sleep, and is available in many forms. It may lower blood sugar, so if you have diabetes, discuss this with your care provider.

- DHEA (Dehydroepiandrosterone) is a hormone that can be synthesized from yams, but is also made by the adrenal gland. It is metabolized into estrogen and testosterone, and has been credited with improving many menopausal symptoms including bone density loss, hot flashes, decreased libido, anxiety, vaginal dryness, and insomnia. Studies have had mixed results for all of these symptoms, and no rigorous randomized studies have yet shown it to be effective for any of them.

You'll find many other herbal compounds and nutritional supplements on grocery and pharmacy shelves. As recommended earlier, do your own research and discuss it with your care provider before you begin using it.

Plant Estrogens

The popular press has played up the use of plant estrogens, called phytohormones, in the treatment of menopausal symptoms.

 Question

What is a bioflavonoid?
Bioflavonoids are naturally occurring plant substances found in many brightly colored fruits and vegetables, such as cherries, oranges and other citrus, grapes, leafy vegetables, wine, and some types of red clover. Researchers are studying bioflavonoids for the treatment of a number of conditions, including the control of bleeding, hemorrhoids, and varicose veins.

Understanding Plant Hormones

So how can a plant or herb compound relieve the symptoms of hormone depletion and imbalance? The answer to that question lies in the chemical makeup of certain plants that contain phytohormones—natural substances found in some herbs and other plants that help to regulate the plant's growth. Though plant and human hormones are very different substances, phytohormones (some types are referred to as phytoestrogens) can bind to the human body's estrogen receptors; phytoestrogens may act like an estrogen on the body or like an anti-estrogen, depending upon the particular type and dosage.

Two of the most popular types of phytoestrogens used in menopausal supplements today are isoflavones (a class of bioflavonoids) and lignans. Isoflavones occur in soybeans, red clover, and (in much lower quantities) green tea, peas, pinto beans, lentils, and other legumes. Lignans occur in flaxseeds (though flaxseed oil contains only small amounts).

Natural estrogen can be extracted from some foods, such as soy; and plant hormones from the wild yam have been extracted to create a progesterone-like cream. Some tests have shown that certain plant estrogens offer some relief from hot flashes of perimenopause and menopause, if the symptoms are mild. They are the subject of a great deal of ongoing research, as the medical community continues to test the safety and efficacy of these substances and to learn how their use compares with the effectiveness of traditional MHT in the treatment of symptoms of women with diminishing levels of hormone production.

 Alert

Studies are constantly changing our understanding of these natural alternatives to MHT. To stay current on the uses of these substances, read information by researchers and clinicians. Use the information you gain in this chapter as a foundation for your own research and discussions with your health care professional.

Soy and Isoflavones

Soy is a major source of a number of important vitamins and nutrients, and it is one of the primary sources for isoflavones—a type of plant estrogen. The North American Menopause Society (NAMS) has reported on a number of studies of the use of isoflavones and their role in managing menopausal health (see Appendix C). Though some of the studies have been inconclusive and work continues in this area, many health and nutrition experts believe that soy has major benefits for treating some symptoms of menopause:

- The isoflavones in soy may help reduce LDL ("bad") cholesterol and triglycerides while increasing HDL ("good") cholesterol levels.
- Many women find that soy reduces the occurrences and the severity of hot flashes.
- One study, reported in 2001, found that women who included whole soy foods in their diet had reductions in some of the key indicators for the onset of osteoporosis. (You can read this study online at *www.menopause.org* under abstract 85384 or see Appendix C for its print source in the NAMS journal.)

- Some women report that an increased intake of soy isoflavones helps alleviate their symptoms of vaginal dryness, though no long-term study has confirmed this.

Keep in mind that the type of soy you consume has a huge impact on the amount of symptom relief you may be able to expect. For example, raw, green soybeans contain the most isoflavones—as much as 150 milligrams per 100 grams of food—whereas soy hot dogs or breakfast sausage may contain only 3 or 4 milligrams. Most medical experts recommend that if you're using soy to manage menopause symptoms that you consume at least 100 milligrams per day (for 25 to 50 milligrams of isoflavones). In the Scheiber NAMS Fellowship study mentioned earlier, the participants ate whole soy foods containing 60 mg/d every day.

Soy products aren't calorie-free, but they tend to be low in fat, high in dietary fiber, and full of vitamins and minerals. Soy milk, tofu, tempeh, and imitation meat products such as burgers, sausage, and "unchicken" cutlets are some of the readily available sources of soy. Soy sprouts, soy flour, and roasted soybeans are also rich sources of soy isoflavones.

 Fact

Asian women, who often eat a diet rich in soy products, have exceptionally low rates of hip and spine fractures and endometrial, breast, and ovarian cancers. Although the Asian diet is also low in red meat and saturated animal fats, researchers are tracking down possible connections between the consumption of soy isoflavones and the low rate of hormone-related conditions.

Red clover is the second richest source of isoflavones. Though some herbal teas and compounds include red clover, it's more commonly taken as a plant extract. There is no clear evidence that red clover is effective in relieving menopausal symptoms, including hot flashes, but the studies do not report serious side effects either. Some animal studies have raised the question about red clover's effect on hormone sensitive tissues such as breast and uterine tissue, but no human studies have looked at this.

Alert

> Scientists are still not clear about how the plant estrogens (phytoestrogens) found in soy and red clover operate in a woman's body. If you have had (or at high risk for) uterine, breast, or ovarian cancer, endometriosis, uterine fibroids, or if you are on hormone therapy, cancer drugs or designer estrogens (SERMs), do not use these substances without first having a serious discussion with your health care provider.

Therapeutic Programs

Women in the United States are learning that many of the medical traditions from other cultures have some use for the management of menopausal symptoms. And some traditional Western therapies such as counseling and cognitive therapy are incredibly effective for treating some of the most debilitating symptoms of menopause, including mood swings, irritability, and depression.

So Many Therapies, So Little Time

If you want to turn to a more holistic approach, there are plenty from which to choose. Depending on whether you prefer to work through your body or your mind—although the two obviously impact each other!—there are approaches that can help you manage many of your current life challenges, menopause being just one.

The following list discusses some of the therapeutic programs that women have found useful in treating symptoms of perimenopause and menopause:

- Acupuncture is an ancient Chinese therapy that involves rotating fine needles until they enter the skin at specific points on the body. In a 1995 test reported by the North American Menopause Society (NAMS) in the journal Menopause, women treated with both electrically aided and traditional acupuncture showed a significant decrease in hot flashes, lasting up to three months after treatment. Other studies have shown acupuncture to decrease the severity of nighttime hot flashes (thus improving sleep quality) and to decrease anxiety in menopausal women. The National Institute of Health Consensus Development Panel on Acupuncture issued a statement saying that acupuncture may be helpful in managing conditions such as headache, fibromyalgia, osteoarthritis, and cramps—conditions some women face in perimenopause and menopause.

- Breathing regulation, where women are trained to breathe deeply and slowly (sometimes called paced respiration), has also shown some promise in reducing hot flashes and aiding relaxation. For perimenopausal and menopausal women suffering from hot flashes, anxiety, and panic attacks, this technique can be particularly useful. Perhaps due to the same calm, slow respiratory technique taught in practices such as yoga and meditation, some women report those practices have also helped them to alleviate anxiety as well as the frequency and intensity of hot flashes.

 Fact

Many women claim to have found real relief from hot flashes, anxiety, and other menopausal symptoms through acupressure and therapeutic massage. In acupressure, a therapist places pressure on the body at the same meridian points used in acupuncture. Many types of therapeutic massage operate on the principle that stimulating the body's circulation and lymph gland production boosts health.

- Biofeedback is a technique in which individuals are trained to monitor bodily functions such as breathing, heart rate, and blood pressure, and then change those functions through relaxation techniques or visual imagery. Studies on biofeedback have been ongoing since the 1970s, and some have indicated that biofeedback techniques can help women control hot flashes and stress urinary incontinence.

- Cognitive therapy—a type of talk therapy—focuses on helping the individual learn to see the connection between a pattern of negative thought and depression. As you learn to replace negative thoughts with positive ones, you can break damaging thinking patterns that contribute to deepening, ongoing depression, and anxiety.

Keep Your Eyes on the Prize

As you approach menopause, you may find that you gain a greater appreciation every day of your health and its precious gifts. But as the medical profession uncovers new treatment strategies, what people know about menopause evolves. As you evaluate and follow treatment options for maintaining your physical and emotional health throughout this time in your life, remember to keep an open mind and remain curious.

Essential

The real prize in menopause is the chance to regain or retain your healthy body so that it can carry you into your third age with comfort and vitality. Every choice you make moves you either toward or away from this goal. Understanding all the choices helps you make conscious decisions to stay healthy well beyond your menopause.

Follow medical developments, closely monitor your symptoms and treatment reactions, and continue to work with your health care provider to make sure that the plan you've chosen is the best option for you today. Nothing stays the same, and you can't assume that today's treatment decision will still be the best choice throughout all of your tomorrows.

CHAPTER 13

Health Risks after Forty

IF THE FIRST FORTY YEARS of your life were spent in blissful ignorance of the toll that each passing year might take on your physical health, now is the time to get serious about a personal maintenance plan. If you are aware of the common health risks women face after forty, you will know what changes you need to make in your diet and lifestyle. This chapter will summarize these risks.

The Health Risks You Face after Forty

Introducing you to health risks is not saying that turning forty some-how signals an onslaught of diseases and disabilities. Many women are healthier than they've ever been as they approach midlife. But a well-thought-out approach to health maintenance is smart at any age, and it becomes more important as each year passes. Don't think of your health care efforts as part of entering old age; think of them as a simple, basic plan to preserve and extend your energy and quality of life.

Time for a Tune-Up?

Everyone—man and woman—has to invest a bit more time and attention in his or her "machine" as it ages. Your body works hard, and after years of service even routine maintenance becomes more demand-ing—and essential. You lose track of the tradeoffs you've made in how you spend your time and mental energy with less time spent outdoors moving your body, and more time spent sitting behind a desk or in the car, struggling to meet deadlines, resolving problems, or sorting out schedules. Many people enter their forties wedged between caring for their children and their parents. Add to that the accumulation of many years of not-so-healthy habits and it's easy to see why your body might need a little TLC as it hits midlife.

As Estrogen Wanes

Estrogen provides women with a natural protection against certain diseases, such as osteoporosis, high cholesterol, and vaginal atrophy. In perimenopause, a woman's body produces less estrogen, making her more vulnerable to these and other health risks. Many physical symptoms that might be attributed to the first pangs of aging might actually be the first warning signals of serious health problems. So a good health care regimen at age forty can lay the groundwork for a healthy passage through ages fifty, sixty, seventy, eighty, and beyond.

⌷ Essential

Many women view breast cancer as their greatest health threat, but heart disease is a much greater risk for women. According to the American Heart Association (AHA), nearly twice as many women in the United States die of heart disease and stroke than from all forms of cancer combined—and that includes breast cancer.

Heart Disease

You've probably heard, but may not fully understand, the term "heart disease." The umbrella term covers a wide range of diseases, illnesses, and events—known as cardiovascular diseases—that impact the heart and circulatory system. High blood pressure and coronary artery disease that can lead to stroke, heart attacks, and early death are some of the most common forms of heart disease for both men and women.

High Blood Pressure

For reasons that aren't entirely clear, women seem to lose their natural "protection" from cardiovascular disease when their estrogen begins to wane. Sometimes the first sign of this is a rise in blood pressure, also known as hypertension. When your blood pressure rises and stays elevated, it can lead to stroke, heart attack, or kidney failure. Sometimes this change happens slowly and the numbers creep up over time. Sometimes, for no apparent reason, a woman will suddenly have very high blood pressure. Menopause is the perfect time to begin tracking your blood pressure, in case you are one of the 35 million women who have high blood pressure.

Heart Attack

A heart attack, also known as myocardial infarction, happens when one of your arteries is blocked, keeping the heart from getting the blood it needs. Until recently, much of the research on cardiovascular disease was done on men, and the "classic" symptoms of a heart attack were not necessarily the same ones women experience. While women have a lower incidence of heart attacks than men until age forty-five, it quickly evens out. In later years, women surpass men in their risk of myocardial infarction. See Chapter 14 for more information on heart attacks in women.

Stroke

A stroke refers to damage in the brain caused by either a bleeding into the brain, or when a blood vessel to the brain is blocked and brain tissue does not get oxygen and nutrients. This damage to the brain can cause death or serious disability. Women are more likely than men to have a stroke, and more than 60 percent of stroke deaths are women. You are at higher risk for stroke as you get past forty-five, and in particular if you are a smoker, have a family history of stroke, or have untreated high blood pressure.

 Fact

If you're courting obesity and high cholesterol, you're speeding up the effects of age on your heart. According to the American Heart Association's 2001 Heart and Stroke Statistical Update, nearly 34 percent of the average diet in the United States is made up of fat and over half of all Americans have high blood total cholesterol levels (over 200 mg/dl or milligrams per deciliter of blood).

High Cholesterol

Cholesterol is a waxy sort of fat that is circulated in your bloodstream. Natural estrogen in your system prior to menopause seems to keep the "good" cholesterol (HDL) high, and the "bad" cholesterol (LDL) low. Once estrogen declines, this reverses and these fatty substances begin to block blood vessels in the same way they do in men. Women over forty-five have the same risk for high cholesterol as men, and begin to suffer from heart disease at the same rate. Chapter 14 has more information on cholesterol and ways to minimize its impact on your health. If you are over forty-five, get a baseline cholesterol test so you can monitor it over the next years.

Cancer Risks

Though heart disease is a more common disease among American women, cancer is one of the most feared. Cancer is the second leading cause of death in the United States; nearly four of every ten Americans will have some kind of cancer at some point during their lives, and about 75 percent of those diagnosed with cancer are age fifty-five or older. One-third of all women in the United States will develop cancer during their lifetimes, so as you approach menopause, it's important that you understand which cancers have age-related risk factors for women.

Cancer isn't one disease, but a family of diseases, all of which occur when cell growth goes out of control in some part of the body. Contributing factors include environmental pollutants, heredity, occupation, nutrition, and lifestyle. Different cancers produce very different illnesses, each with its own symptoms, causes, and risk factors. The following sections discuss some of the most common cancers women face as they move into middle age.

Lung Cancer

Lung cancer is the leading cause of cancer death for women in the United States, and tobacco smoke is the leading cause of lung cancer. Though neither menopause nor age is a contributing factor in this disease, most women are diagnosed with lung cancer at age fifty—right around the time they hit menopause, and often after many years of tobacco smoke exposure. Women are one and a half times as likely as men to develop cancer from tobacco smoke, including secondhand smoke; the vast majority of nonsmokers who contract lung cancer are women.

 ## Alert

Since 1950, lung cancer deaths in women in the United States have increased by a startling 600 percent. Every woman smoker knows she should quit, but many fear weight gain, anxiety, and unquench-able cravings during withdrawal. If you are a smoker, you have more options for quitting now than ever before, including patches, gum, medications, and hypnosis. Do whatever it takes to quit now.

Why not start this new phase smoke-free? Smoking increases your chances of developing cervical cancer, emphysema, and other life-threatening chronic lung conditions. Smoking is a sure way to derail an active, healthy passage into middle life. In fact, smokers tend to have earlier menopause than nonsmokers, so quitting early can delay meno-pause in some women.

Breast Cancer

Breast cancer is the second most common form of cancer for American women, and advancing age appears to be a major risk factor in its development. Nearly 80 percent of all breast cancers are found in women over fifty, and the incidence of diagnosis and fatality both seem to rise with age. The American Cancer Society (ACS) reports that 163 per 100,000 women in the United States in their forties are diagnosed with breast cancer each year, and 29 die of it; 374 per 100,000 women in their sixties will be diagnosed, and 90 of those will die from the disease.

If your mother, sister, or daughter has had breast cancer, your risks of getting it go up two to three times (depending on how many of these first-degree relatives are involved). And, if you've had breast cancer before, you have a higher risk of developing it again. If you've never had a child, or had your first child after age thirty, your risk goes up as well. But what about risk factors that you can change? The ACS lists the following risk factors for breast cancer that are specifically linked to lifestyle choices:

- **Menopause hormone therapy.** MHT does appear to increase the risk of certain types of breast cancer in some women. In 2006, it was reported that after the Women's Health Initiative (WHI) study results were made public, millions of women stopped MHT. The following year, the incidence of breast cancers, especially estrogen-sensitive breast cancers, had dropped by 7 percent. This is the largest drop in breast cancer rates since records were first kept in the 1970s. This strongly suggests a link between MHT and breast cancer.

  In the Nurses Health Study of 121,700 women patients, those using estrogen alone had a 23 percent increase in breast cancer over women who never used hormone therapy. Estrogen with progesterone was even more concerning, with a 58 percent increased risk of breast cancer. The most alarming was the 77 percent higher risk for women taking estrogen plus testosterone. Based on these results as well as the WHI study, it would be fair to say that using any sort of MHT has a chance of increasing your breast cancer risk.

- **Alcohol.** Women who have one alcoholic drink a day have a slightly increased risk of contracting breast cancer; two to five drinks daily can up your risk to one-and-a-half times that of nondrinkers.

- **Diet.** The connection between obesity and breast cancer risk is still being studied, but research indicates that after menopause your risk of contracting breast cancer is greater if you are overweight. How much of this risk is linked to your body fat versus specific dietary fat content is still not clear. Another issue may be that more breast tissue (obese women tend to have bigger breasts) makes it harder to find an early, small cancerous lump, both on exam and on mammogram.

- **Exercise.** Although research has begun only recently, early findings reported by the ACS seem to indicate that even moderate physical activity can lower breast cancer risk. And maintaining good overall physical condition certainly improves your chances of having fewer complications related to medical and surgical treatment for any disease—including breast cancer.

Survival rates for breast cancer are highest when the cancer is detected early. The five-year survival rate (your chance of being alive five years after the diagnosis of cancer is made) is 96 percent for women whose cancer is caught at an early stage. Early detection helps keep the surgery or other treatment that follows diagnosis as noninvasive and conservative as is possible. Techniques for incorporating breast cancer detection into your general health maintenance plan appear later in this chapter.

Endometrial Cancer

In the United States, cancer of the endometrium—the lining of the uterus—is the most common cancer of the female reproductive organs. The ACS estimates that this cancer has a five-year survival rate of about 84 percent.

Your risk of developing endometrial cancer increases as you age. The average age of diagnosis for this cancer is sixty, and 95 percent of all endometrial cancer occurs in women age forty or older.

 Fact

Endometrial cancer is usually preceded by a precancerous condition called endometrial hyperplasia, which is easily diagnosed with a test—endometrial biopsy—that your physician can perform in the office. This test takes about one minute, requires no anesthesia or sedation, and produces very reliable results.

A number of risk factors can contribute to the development of endometrial cancer:

- **Total number of years of anovulatory cycles.** Your body's total lifetime exposure to estrogen, without the balancing hormone progesterone, can have an impact on your likelihood of developing endometrial cancer. The more cycles you have had without ovulation, the more you have been exposed to unopposed estrogen, and the higher your risk. If you began having periods at a young age (before the age of twelve), continued having periods past age fifty, and have had few or no children (which gives your body a break from the constant estrogen production), your ovaries have been producing estrogen for a greater number of years than the average woman. The more estrogen (and less progesterone) your body has experienced over the years, the higher your risk of developing endometrial cancer.

- **Obesity.** Depending upon how obese you are, your excess body fat can increase your chances of developing endometrial cancer two to five times. Body fat can convert other hormones into estrogen, and having excess body fat contributes to a woman's estrogen levels—and risks of developing this cancer. Diets high in animal fats also may contribute to this risk factor, as can diabetes—a disease common among obese women. Women who are overweight are also more likely to have abnormal menstrual periods, because their ovaries fail to ovulate—thus not producing enough progesterone to balance their estrogen.

- **Estrogen therapy (ET).** ET—hormone therapy that doesn't include progesterone—can increase a woman's chance of developing endometrial cancer. Though doctors used to prescribe ET for relief from hot flashes, osteoporosis, and heart disease, today doctors almost exclusively combine estrogen with progesterone in MHT, which eliminates the increased risk of endometrial cancer. Of course, if you have had a hysterectomy, you do not need a prescription for progesterone added to your estrogen, since your risk of endometrial cancer is zero.

Alert

Pap smears are not enough. Pap smears—which are great at detecting cervical cancer—don't reveal endometrial cancer. A normal pap smear is not a clean bill of health. Unless you're at high risk for developing this disease, your doctor won't routinely order yearly detection tests. Talk to your care provider about whether you are at risk for endometrial cancer, and whether tests should be run.

If endometrial cancer is diagnosed early, it has an excellent survival rate. Precancerous changes, such as endometrial hyperplasia, often become known through unusual spotting, bleeding, or discharge. Often, these symptoms are apparent for years before actual cancer develops. Sometimes women who have had irregular periods for their entire lives forget to report this to their health care practitioner. Besides, when you're entering menopause, irregular bleeding, spotting, and discharges aren't supposed to be unusual occurrences at all, so how do you know when to worry that your irregularity is signaling endometrial cancer?

If you suffer from unusual bleeding that lasts more than two weeks, consult your doctor right away—no matter what your medical history. An endometrial biopsy can determine whether or not your symptoms point to endometrial cancer or some other cause.

Ovarian Cancer

One in 70 women will develop ovarian cancer over the course of her life; it's the fourth leading cause of cancer deaths in women in the United States. Every year, U.S. doctors diagnose over 23,000 cases of this cancer, and more than 14,000 women die from it. Ovarian cancer occurs most often in women who are approaching the age of menopause. This cancer is a silent killer with symptoms that can be mild, vague, and similar to those of many other conditions and diseases. If detected early, while still in the ovary (called stage I), this cancer is curable about 90 percent of the time. But if the cancer spreads to the pelvis or beyond (stage III or IV), the five-year survival rate drops dramatically. Taking all stages into consideration, this cancer's overall five-year survival rate is somewhere around 40 percent.

Fact

If you have had breast, colon, or ovarian cancer, you may have an increased risk for developing endometrial cancer. Some of the same risk factors contribute to all of these forms of cancer, so with the diagnosis of one, your physician will also monitor you closely for these other cancer types.

Sadly, early ovarian cancer has few symptoms, so it makes sense to know your risk factors and your family history. Risk factors for ovarian cancer include:

- A family history of ovarian, breast, colon, rectal, endometrial, or pancreatic cancer increases a woman's risks considerably. The severity of increased risk is higher if there has been one of these cancers in a first-degree relative, such as a mother, sister, or daughter.
- A woman's risk of developing ovarian cancer also rises with the total number of times she has ovulated; again, exposure to estrogen has an impact on the woman's overall risks. In other words, not having had any children or not taking birth control pills at any point in your life means your ovaries have been working overtime, compared to women in the average population.

Symptoms of ovarian cancer are vague, especially in the early stage, but can include pain, pressure, or swelling in your abdomen; gas, nausea, and indigestion; unexplained changes in your bowel movements; changes in your weight; fatigue; or pain during intercourse. If you exhibit any of these symptoms, talk to your doctor. He or she can perform a sonogram (ultrasound examination of the pelvis) to determine if your ovaries have any abnormalities. In addition, your health care provider may choose to obtain a blood test called CA-125 to check for a certain protein that can point to the presence of ovarian tumors. It is not a perfect test. A negative result does not rule out ovarian cancer, since about half of tests are negative in stage I of the disease; an elevated result does not always mean ovarian cancer—it can point to liver problems, colon conditions such as diverticulitis, and other illnesses. Inaccurate results with this blood test (a false positive) are highest in premenopausal women, so check with your doctor about the usefulness of taking the test and with your insurance company about whether it is covered.

Of course, your health care provider physically palpates (feels) your ovaries every year during your pelvic examination to detect any changes in their size or shape. In most cases, a combination of symptoms and physical examination findings lead to a series of diagnostic tests for ovarian cancer. That's why now, more than ever, it's critical that you report any unusual physical symptoms or changes in your normal menstrual cycle to your health care provider.

Question

What should I do if I think I might have ovarian cancer?
Contact your health care provider or see a gynecologist. To learn more about this disease call the National Cancer Institute's Cancer Information Service (CIS) at 800-4-CANCER (800-422-6237) or visit its ovarian cancer information Web site at *www.cancer .gov/cancertopics/types/ovarian.*

Osteoporosis

Osteoporosis—the loss of bone mass that results in porous, fragile bones—threatens nearly 28 million people in the United States, 80 percent of whom are women. According to the National Osteoporosis Foundation, 8 million women have osteoporosis and millions more have low bone density. Half of all women over the age of fifty will suffer an osteoporosis-related bone fracture at some time during their lives. Most of these fractures are preventable if a doctor diagnoses the early stages of osteoporosis, called osteopenia, at a time when preventable measures are possible. Bone wellness is discussed in detail in Chapter 15, Maintaining Bone Health.

⌶ Essential

Don't overlook the importance of getting a bone density screening test! Osteopenia—early bone loss not severe enough to qualify as osteoporosis but a definite warning sign—is present in over two-thirds of the population of women. These statistics have emerged only recently, as bone density screening tests have become more common.

Urinary Tract Disorders and Yeast Infections

During perimenopause, about 40 percent of women experience some form of urogenital changes—changes to the vagina, genitals, and urinary tract. Thin, unelastic vaginal tissue is more easily irritated and broken, and therefore more prone to infections such as vaginitis, yeast infections, and urinary tract infections (UTIs). The severity of these disorders ranges from mildly irritating to very painful.

Vaginitis

Most women have experienced some type of vaginitis (a swollen, red, irritated vaginal area) at some point in life. These infections include bacterial vaginosis, yeast infections, and trichomoniasis. During perimenopause, fluctuating hormone levels can contribute to the frequency and severity of these infections. Bacteria in the vagina, obesity, diabetes, and antibiotics are other contributors. The symptoms of these vaginal infections include burning and itching in the vaginal area and a discharge.

If you've had yeast infections before and are relatively certain that you're suffering from this type of infection, you can use any of the available over-the-counter creams and other treatments. But if you experience new or unusual symptoms, or the symptoms continue or recur (especially after using an over-the-counter medication), see your physician for a full diagnosis and treatment. And although you can't prevent all vaginal infections, here are some ways to try to avoid them:

- Don't wear tight clothes (such as jeans) that block air circulation to your lower body, and don't wear underpants to bed at night.
- Wear underwear and pantyhose with cotton crotches (avoid pantyhose if you can).
- Be clean; wash your genital area thoroughly, front to back, every day.
- Stay away from heavily perfumed and deodorizing soaps, douches, sprays, tampons, and pads, and use white unscented toilet paper. All of those perfumes and deodorant chemicals can dry out your skin and contribute to acid-level imbalances in your vagina that can lead to infections.

Fewer layers of clothing are better than too many (though layering the clothes on your upper body is a good idea when you suffer from hot flashes); looser is better than too tight; and natural fabrics such as cotton are better than spandex and other "unbreathable" blends. After exercising, swimming, or otherwise working up a sweat, change out of sweaty clothes and get into something clean and dry.

 Fact

If vaginal dryness is a problem for you, your doctor might recommend more frequent sex as a treatment! Sexual arousal—even from masturbation—is a great way to help keep your vaginal tissues moist and flexible and stave off the effects of vaginal atrophy.

Urinary Tract Infections

Urinary tract infections (UTIs) are common in women of all ages, but can be particularly persistent following menopause. In addition to the susceptibility of thin, dry vaginal tissue to infection, the lactobacilli organisms that help fight off bacterial infections in the vagina decline after menopause. And, as the bladder muscles weaken with age, the bladder doesn't empty completely, which can contribute to the buildup of bacteria. UTIs, including cystitis (bladder infection) and urethritis (infection in the urethra), are caused by bacteria (usually from skin around the anus) traveling through the urethra and reaching the bladder, or even the kidneys. These bacteria trigger infections that result in symptoms such as pain or burning during urination; sudden, strong, and frequent urges to urinate; fever and chills; and even pain in your back, side, or abdomen.

If you have painful urination, accompanied by pain in your back and fever, you may have a kidney infection. Kidney infections can result in chronic and even life-threatening consequences if untreated, so call your doctor immediately if you have these symptoms. Again, these infections can grow much worse if untreated, so you need to contact your doctor if you experience them. Sometimes more than one course of antibiotics or a different type of antibiotic is necessary to eradicate the bacteria completely.

If recurrent UTIs or symptoms that resemble UTIs become a problem for you, your doctor or health care provider might recommend estrogen cream or MHT to help rejuvenate your vaginal tissue. The estrogen helps increase the blood circulation to this area and restores natural secretions, thus making the entire vagina and urinary tract less susceptible to injury and infection. But you might be able to avoid some of these infections or discomforts through some simple, healthy habits:

- Wipe from front to back, so you don't push bacteria from your anus over your vaginal tissue.
- Drink lots of fluids (water is best) and urinate frequently to keep your urethra (the opening to the bladder) flushed out.
- Practice clean, safe sex, and always urinate after sex to flush bacteria from your urethra. It's a good idea for both partners to wash hands and genitals before having sex.
- Use a water-based lubricant (rather than an oil-based product such as petroleum jelly) to reduce friction during sex.

Assessing Your Health History

Everyone tells you that you inherited your father's temper and your mother's beautiful smile, but what else did your parents and grandparents hand down to you? Knowing your family's medical history is one of the best tools you have for predicting your future health. Many of the health risks that deserve your attention as you approach the age of menopause have risk factors associated with your personal health history and the health history of your immediate family. Your doctor or health care provider will want and need to know this information in order to monitor your health, prescribe appropriate treatment, and recommend appropriate preventative measures. Though this information is always important to your health care provider, it becomes essential as you enter perimenopause. If you have children, this information is important to them as well.

Start Asking Questions

Most health care providers ask you to fill out a health history during your first appointment. If you aren't well versed in the medical history of your parents, grandparents, and siblings, talk to your family members ahead of time to gather this information. You'll want to gather medical information about as many of your family members as possible, but remember that your immediate family matters most. You can draw up your own form, fill it in for each family member, and take the forms with you to your medical appointment. For each family member, you should list the name, sex, relationship to you, year of birth, and year and cause of death. Then, note whether that person was ever diagnosed with any of the following health problems:

- alcoholism
- allergies
- Alzheimer's
- angina
- breast cancer
- cervical cancer
- colon cancer

- coronary bypass surgery
- depression
- diabetes
- emphysema
- endometrial cancer
- heart attack
- heart disease

- high blood pressure
- high cholesterol
- lung cancer
- miscarriages, stillbirths, or other problems in pregnancy
- obesity

- osteoporosis
- other cancer (list)
- ovarian cancer
- schizophrenia or other psychiatric disorders (list)
- stroke

If members of your immediate family died at an early age from medical conditions (not accidental deaths), you should also ask other family members about those individuals' lifestyles and living conditions. Did they smoke or drink excessively? Did their jobs or living environment expose them to potentially toxic substances? Did they seem to be under a great deal of stress, or were there any other factors that might have contributed to an early death? The more you—and your doctor—know about the health problems that your relatives have experienced, the better able you'll be to develop a lifestyle and health maintenance plan to help protect you from inherited risks.

Don't Forget Your Own History

Your doctor or health care professional will want to know the same information about you that you've gathered about your family members. Your medical history form will also ask about what illnesses, diseases, surgeries, hospitalizations, and other health issues you've experienced. Gather the information before your doctor's appointment, so you're fully prepared to discuss your history. Try to remember (or better yet, write down) dates of surgeries and hospitalizations. If you've taken birth control pills prescribed by another doctor, write down the brand name and the dates during which you took them. If you are tracking your menopausal symptoms on a menstrual calendar, bring that along as well.

CHAPTER 14

Menopause and Heart Disease

THOUGH IT'S THE number one killer of American women today, few women would name heart disease as a major health concern. The problems that contribute to heart disease can grow silently over a number of years. Even the first signs of serious heart illness, such as a heart attack or stroke, can be attributed to other causes and therefore go unrecognized. This chapter will discuss the symptoms of heart disease, its links to menopause, and how you can control your risks.

What Is Heart Disease?

The term heart disease refers to any disorder or condition of the heart and blood vessels; these diseases fall under the catchall category of cardiovascular disease. Coronary artery disease is a common form of heart disease that occurs when arteries become lined with heavy deposits of plaque—a substance made up of fat, calcium, and other minerals. The plaque buildup narrows the diameter of the vessels, thus limiting the amount of blood that can flow through the arteries, contributing to a condition known as atherosclerosis. As plaque narrows or blocks the coronary arteries, the heart is starved of oxygen, which can lead to a heart attack—and damage the heart muscle itself.

Other heart diseases include congestive heart failure, diseases of the heart valves, irregular heartbeats (arrhythmias), and congenital heart diseases. But for women entering menopause, the threat of heart disease comes mainly from coronary artery disease, the atherosclerosis that contributes to it, and the heart attacks and stroke that all of these conditions can lead to.

Fact

Atherosclerosis can also contribute to the plaque buildup in the carotid arteries that carry oxygen-rich blood to the brain. The plaque buildup can lead to the formation of blood clots, which can break loose from the inside of the vessel walls and be carried to your brain, causing a stroke. In 2003, 96,200 women died of stroke.

The Symptoms of Heart Disease

Unfortunately, coronary artery disease can reach an advanced state without ever issuing a warning sign or symptom. The first major symptom you're likely to experience is a chest pain called angina—a squeezing, heaviness, or tightness in your chest that happens when your heart is starved of oxygen. You might feel this pain when you're exercising, climbing stairs, or rushing to a meeting, or when you're feeling stressed out or highly emotional. At first, the feeling may be just a momentary pressure that passes quickly if you stop and rest for a moment. However, as the arteries become narrower, you're likely to feel the pain again, and it may radiate down your left arm and shoulder, up through your neck and jaw, or down your back. As the atherosclerosis progresses, the pain of angina can become worse. Angina is one warning that you have heart disease and are at risk for suffering a heart attack.

On the other hand, you may have no warning at all. Many people are unaware that they suffer from any kind of heart disease until they have a heart attack, but women are more likely than men to experience the warning pangs of angina before a full heart attack occurs. Because the symptoms of angina are very much like those of a heart attack, it's critical that you report those symptoms to your health care provider immediately for diagnosis.

When a Heart Attack Hits

If one or more of your coronary arteries become completely blocked, you can have a heart attack. Over 200,000 women die of heart attack every year in this country, and almost 20,000 of them are under sixty-five. Many thousands more suffer an attack and survive. A heart attack can be mild, moderate, or severe, depending upon the amount of damage to the heart muscle. If only a small area of the heart is deprived of blood, the healthy heart tissue surrounding it continues to work, allowing the damaged part of the heart to heal as new vessels grow in from the healthy areas. But if damage occurs in several of these small areas, they can combine to damage the heart beyond repair.

The symptoms of heart attack vary; in some cases, the attack is so minor that no noticeable symptoms occur. In fact, women may have very different symptoms than men, and heart attacks in women are misdiagnosed as other conditions such as anxiety and indigestion. With careful attention, though, heart attack symptoms can be recognized and women can seek treatment. Those symptoms include the following:

- A crushing or dull pain in the chest
- Pain in the left shoulder, arm, neck, or back
- Nausea, vomiting
- Difficulty breathing
- Fatigue or dizziness
- Burning pain in the middle chest area or upper abdomen area similar to heartburn or indigestion
- Profuse sweating

And pay special attention to these unusual symptoms that may signal a heart attack for women, and are uncommon in men:

- Weakness or profound fatigue
- Light-headedness
- Fainting
- Sudden or extreme anxiety or a "feeling of doom"

Alert

> According to the American Medical Association (AMA), as many as one-third of heart attacks go undiagnosed in women—or are attributed to some other cause, such as indigestion. If you have any of the symptoms of a heart attack, contact your doctor immediately.

You Are Your Own "First Responder"

Only rarely do heart attacks cause the heart to stop functioning completely. More often, you have a chance to make a big difference in the amount of damage your heart receives and your chances for a recovery. But you must act quickly; most heart attack damage occurs within the first two hours after you feel the pain. If you have any reason to suspect you may be having an attack—a personal history of angina or a family history of heart disease—be prepared to get help. Sit or lie down for a minute or two. If you continue to feel the symptoms, call an ambulance or 911 and tell the operator you might be having a heart attack. Then, follow that operator's instructions until the ambulance arrives. For example, the operator is likely to ask you to take an aspirin as you wait for the paramedics.

If you have the symptoms of heart attack, don't drive yourself to the hospital and don't avoid calling for help because you aren't certain the pains you feel are a heart attack. If there was ever a situation in which the old "better safe than sorry" expression applies, this is it. Be smart. Get medical attention immediately.

Women, Menopause, and Heart Disease

Now that you know what heart disease is, you might be wondering why you need to be concerned about it now. After all, if you're just entering perimenopause, you're probably in your forties, or if you've just experienced menopause, you might be in your early fifties. You're far from some old-timer who needs to worry about a failing heart—right?

Actually, you're right about the first part of that statement, but wrong about the last. At forty or fifty, you're far from being an old-timer, but heart disease doesn't strike only the elderly. Heart disease is the number one killer of women age fifty and over. One in five women has some type of heart or blood vessel disease, and every year nearly half a million women in the United States die from cardiovascular diseases.

Women in their childbearing years are less prone to heart disease than are men of the same age. However, according to the American Heart Association (AHA), "Menopause itself appears to increase a woman's risks of coronary heart disease and stroke." Your risk of heart disease increases when you reach menopause—then just keeps on increasing. If your menopause occurs naturally, the risk rises slowly. But if menopause results from surgery, the risks can rise dramatically and quickly.

Essential

From 1999 to 2003 the number of women dying from cardiovascular disease decreased by 5.7 percent. But in every year since 1984, more women than men have died of heart disease, partly because women are more difficult to diagnose and partly because women are not as likely to get appropriate treatment following a first heart attack.

What's Menopause Got to Do with It?

If women have less risk of heart disease before menopause than do men of the same age, with the same contributing risk factors, why does their postmenopausal risk surpass that of men? To understand this surge in risk, it's important to understand some of the root causes of heart disease in any individual. Though later sections of this chapter discuss these risk factors in detail, one of the most important contributors to heart disease is high blood cholesterol levels. When you develop high blood cholesterol levels, you have too much artery-clogging fat in your bloodstream. The diminished supply of estrogen that occurs with menopause, weight gain, and the aging of your cardiovascular system all contribute to developing high cholesterol levels.

Does Menopause Hormone Therapy Lower Your Risk?

A number of medical researchers and scientists believe that a woman's own natural estrogen might help protect her from heart disease, but they're still studying how the hormone may have that effect. Estrogen plays an important role in maintaining healthy, strong muscle tissue, including the muscle of the heart. Estrogen also has an impact on the blood's level of triglycerides and low-density lipoproteins (LDL) or "bad" cholesterol, both of which can contribute to atherosclerosis and heart attack. Some studies have shown that estrogen contributes to healthy, reactive arteries and an increased blood flow. As a result, blood vessels are better able to relax and respond to exercise and physical stress by dilating and providing more blood flow when needed.

 Fact

The American Heart Association (AHA) recommends not placing women on menopause hormone therapy for the sole purpose of preventing or treating cardiovascular disease. While it may be effective for other symptoms, it has not been proven effective in reducing heart disease in postmenopausal women, and may actually increase their risk.

Does that mean that you can avoid heart disease through estrogen or other hormone therapies? Not necessarily. As we learned with the Women's Health Initiative (WHI) study described in Chapter 11, women on some types of hormone therapy may actually have an increased risk of heart disease, stroke, and blood clots. Analysis of another study, The Harvard Nurses Health Study, showed that beginning estrogen therapy very soon after menopause does seem to offer some protection from cardiovascular disease, but starting it ten years or more following menopause does not offer that protection.

Are Women Really Different From Men?

The answer to this is yes, yes, yes! Women are more likely to die of their heart attacks and strokes than men are, even though men have more of these events. Here are some of the differences:

- **Women minimize their cardiac symptoms.** Women seem to "tough it out" more than men, and studies show that when men and women have the same severity of heart disease, women rate it as "mild to moderate" while men rated theirs as "severe." This keeps women from getting the quick and thorough follow-up care they need.

- **Women can have different symptoms than men.** Women sometimes have only anxiety, or a "doomed" feeling; may be "suddenly very tired"; may vomit; or may have burning abdominal pain. Since these are not the symptoms people think of for a heart attack, they put off getting to the hospital.

- **Women may have a condition called "coronary microvascular syndrome."** In this condition, plaque forms evenly in their arteries, and blockages do not show on diagnostic tests. But the artery walls are still blocked at the microscopic level, thus leaving them at risk for a heart attack.

Essential

Women who have symptoms of a heart attack and whose diagnostic studies show no blockage in their arteries should also be screened with the Duke Activity Status Index. This twelve-item questionnaire asks patients to report whether they can perform a number of daily activities without problems. If they respond that they can't do these activities, then the doctor can order further testing to rule out microvascular syndrome.

Risk Factors You Can't Change

As with most serious health conditions, heart disease is rarely the product of a single event or factor. Heart disease has long been the focus of intense medical study, contributing to the knowledge about the many illnesses and conditions that can contribute to its development. Some risk factors are yours for life—risks associated with your age, sex, race, and genetic inheritance—so you have to construct your healthy life plan with the idea that those risks will always be present.

Acknowledge the Odds

The key risk factors for developing heart disease that cannot be controlled are few. Women face the following unchangeable risks for developing heart disease:

- **Gender.** You can't do a thing about your gender. When it comes to heart disease, being a woman has its advantages when you are younger. But those advantages evaporate after menopause, and you begin to have the same risks as your male counterparts.
- **Growing older.** The older you get, the greater your risk for developing heart disease. Four out of five people who die of heart disease are sixty-five or older. And the older women are when they suffer a heart attack, the more likely they are to die of it.
- **Heredity.** If your parents had heart disease, you're more likely to develop it. Sometimes it is because of a propensity to high cholesterol levels. Race-associated conditions can have an impact on heart disease risk, as well. African Americans, Mexican Americans, Native Americans, Asian Americans, and native Hawaiians have a higher risk for developing the disease.
- **Personal history.** If you have already had a heart attack or been diagnosed with heart disease, then your risk is higher than that of other women your age. While you can't change your history, you can be aware of it when you are making health and lifestyle decisions.

Having these unchangeable risk factors doesn't mean you're destined to suffer from heart disease. Consider it a word to the wise if you are aware of fixed risk factors, and then concentrate on the ones that you can influence. Tendency is not destiny, and there are plenty of things you can do to minimize the dangers to your health.

Risks You Can Influence

Once you understand what might make you predisposed to heart disease, you can concentrate on all the ways to minimize the other risk factors. There are many things you can do to reduce or postpone your chances of developing heart disease.

High Cholesterol

High blood cholesterol is a major risk factor for developing heart disease. After menopause, women tend to develop high levels of triglycerides (a form of fat), in addition to high levels of low-density lipoprotein (LDL), cholesterol. At the same time, their levels of high-density lipoprotein (HDL) can diminish. All of these factors lead to out-of-balance blood cholesterol levels, too much fat in the bloodstream, and the buildup of artery-clogging plaque in the pathways that channel oxygen-rich blood to the heart and brain. For every 1 percent reduction in elevated blood cholesterol levels, you get a 2 to 3 percent reduction in your chances of having a heart attack.

Don't misunderstand the issue about cholesterol; cholesterol is a natural, essential substance in the bloodstream. HDL cholesterol is actually a protein that helps keep all fats and cholesterols moving through your bloodstream (and not glued to your arterial walls), so it actually helps you stave off a potential heart attack. LDL cholesterol moves cholesterol through the rest of your body—but it also has a tendency to linger in your arteries and stick to the walls. Elevated levels of triglycerides may or may not indicate that you're headed for a heart attack, but as another type of fat in the bloodstream, their levels need to be monitored.

So how much is too much (or not enough) of these substances? While your total blood cholesterol level should remain below 180 mg/dl (milligrams per deciliter of blood), and anything over 239 mg/dl needs to be considered a high risk, here's how the individual cholesterol numbers should stack up:

- **HDL:** more than 60 mg/dl is a good number here, less than 40 mg/dl puts you at high risk.
- **LDL:** less than 100 mg/dl is desirable, 130 to 159 mg/dl is considered borderline high, and 160 mg/dl to 189 mg/dl is high risk, with 190 mg/dl very high risk.
- **Triglycerides:** less than 150 mg/dl is considered normal, 150 to 199 mg/dl is borderline high, 200 to 499 mg/dl is high, and over 500 mg/dl is way too high.

A low-fat diet and regular exercise can help most people maintain healthy blood cholesterol levels. Where those efforts fall short, a variety of cholesterol-lowering drugs, called statins, have entered the market over the past several years. Recent studies have shown that these drugs do actually reduce your risk of dying from a heart disease. Although some of these drugs may have side effects, the medications currently on the market are considered safe and effective. Consult your physician; do not rely on a homeopath or other alternative health care if your lipid profile is abnormal.

 Fact

> Triglycerides are a type of fat found in the blood, but more appealing types of this fat include butter, margarine, and vegetable oil. Eating these fats doesn't automatically result in high triglyceride blood levels, however; the partners in crime here seem to be overindulging in alcohol, being overweight, or having diabetes.

High Blood Pressure

High blood pressure (hypertension) is another silent plague of women age fifty-five and over. More than half of all women in that age group have blood pressure greater than 140/90 (the high-blood-pressure threshold), but few of them feel its effects. In fact, though some estimates say that one in four people in the United States suffers from high blood pressure, nearly one-third of those individuals are unaware of their condition. Even if you have had normal blood pressure all of your life, you might develop high blood pressure after menopause. And having high blood pressure makes you a prime candidate for developing heart disease. High blood pressure also contributes to kidney disease and can lead to congestive heart failure, heart attack, and stroke.

 Alert

High blood pressure is a particular threat to African Americans, women over age thirty-five, heavy drinkers, smokers, obese women, and those with diabetes or kidney disease. Blood pressure checks every six months will keep you aware of your own readings so you can seek early treatment if needed.

Like cholesterol, everyone needs blood pressure. After all, blood pressure results from the force of your heart pumping your blood through your veins. If you exercise or become excited, your heart rate increases, sending more blood through your system. If your arteries are clean and wide open, the blood flows freely; if they're narrow or blocked, the buildup of blood trying to course through your veins puts pressure on the arterial walls—and that's high blood pressure. If your arteries are clean and healthy, your blood pressure rises for a short period of time, then returns to normal. If you have hypertension, however, your blood pressure is greater than 135/80–85 even when you're at rest; the extra pressure on your heart and arteries never lets up. If high blood pressure occurs in a person with atherosclerosis, the walls of the vessels are toughened and less elastic, and even less able to cope with stress.

Most doctors consider a blood pressure reading under 120/80 to be ideal. Though some people have suffered from low blood pressure, it's pretty uncommon and not life threatening. Regular exercise and a diet high in vegetables and fruit, but low in sodium, can help control high blood pressure. If diet, exercise, and weight loss (when indicated) don't bring blood pressure down, your health care provider may prescribe drug therapy. Biofeedback and relaxation techniques can also be helpful in keeping your blood pressure down.

Diabetes

Diabetes is another heart disease risk factor that is of particular concern to women. Nearly 6 million women in the United States have been diagnosed with diabetes, and another 2.5 million women have undiagnosed diabetes. Women who have diabetes are at a significantly greater risk of developing heart disease than their non-diabetic "sisters." Having diabetes ups your risk of heart disease and stroke by two to four times. Every year, over 60,000 Americans die of complications of diabetes, and the disease can lead to a host of other conditions, including kidney failure, blindness, and nerve disease.

Diabetes mellitus occurs when the body is unable to produce adequate amounts of insulin or efficiently use the insulin it produces (insulin resistance). Type 2 or adult onset diabetes is the most common form of the disease, and it usually occurs at middle age. Symptoms of diabetes include weight loss, blurred vision, intense thirst, fatigue, excessive urination, and hunger. Doctors test for diabetes through assessing the level of glucose (sugar) in your blood. If a random (non-fasting) glucose screening test is borderline or abnormal, or if your family history is very strong, the doctor may decide to repeat the test. In that test, the doctor may ask you to fast before the first blood sample is taken; then, after you drink a specifically prepared glucose solution, blood samples are taken again at two one-hour intervals. If two of the samples show an elevated blood sugar level, you're considered to be diabetic.

Doctors don't know what causes the development of diabetes, and no drug can cure it. However, diabetes can be controlled—and sometimes disappears altogether—through diet, exercise, and weight loss. Statistics show that 80 to 90 percent of people with diabetes are overweight, and many have high blood pressure and/or lead inactive lives. Though a large number of diabetics require insulin or drug therapy, many others are able to control their disease through behavior modification, such as diet, exercise, and weight loss—a lifelong change that offers big rewards.

⌷ Essential

Obesity

Few conditions are as common and as potentially damaging (both emotionally and physically) as obesity. In fact, obesity has never been more common; the numbers of obese people in the United States continue to rise at alarming levels. The percentage of overweight Americans has risen so dramatically that now nearly two-thirds of all American women are overweight or obese—conditions defined in general by a body weight more than 30 percent over the ideal for the body's height and frame, or having an abnormally high body mass index (BMI). Obesity is damaging in ways few non-obese people can imagine; unlike most other diseases, obesity is commonly viewed as a disease of weakness, self-indulgence, and laziness. Obese people often are the object of ridicule and disdain. Unlike other heart disease risk factors, obesity is plainly visible.

Though obesity can result in obvious emotional distress, its health-damaging effects are even more insidious. Obesity is strongly linked to heart disease in ways that are still under study, but some research indicates that nearly 70 percent of diagnosed cases of heart disease may be directly linked to obesity.

Women are at special risk for heart disease from postmenopausal weight gain. The reason is the location of the added weight; many women tend to add weight in their abdomen and upper body during menopause. This type of fat seems to be linked very closely with a number of other risk factors for heart disease, including diabetes. Because the body's metabolism begins to slow down during perimenopause, you burn fewer calories, even at rest. So if you continue to consume the same number of calories you consumed in your youth, you will almost certainly gain weight.

 Fact

> The link between hypertension and obesity is particularly strong. The American Heart Association (AHA) estimates that over 75 percent of all diagnosed hypertension is directly related to obesity.

Though so many Americans suffer from obesity, researchers are still trying to determine all of the factors that contribute to it. Some contributors are controllable—things such as leading a sedentary lifestyle and consuming a high-fat, high-calorie diet. But if those factors were the only causes of obesity, fewer individuals would suffer from the disease. In fact, gender, age, individual biological and genetic makeup, psychological condition, and environment each appear capable of playing a major role in the development of obesity.

Essential

> High body mass index and waist circumference are both markers of cardiac risk. If your BMI is over 30 (obese) or your waist measures over 35 inches, you are at much higher risk of heart disease than women your age who fall within normal ranges.

Smoking

Smoking tobacco is hard on your entire body, but it delivers a particularly hard blow to your heart. Each time you draw in a lungful of tobacco smoke, you temporarily increase your heart rate and blood pressure and deplete the oxygen in your bloodstream that should be going to feed your heart and other body tissues. If you smoke even one to four cigarettes a day, you're doubling your chances of having a heart attack—and very few smokers smoke four or fewer cigarettes in the average day. Smoke a pack or more, and your risk goes up four times. Over 30 percent of all deaths due to coronary heart disease are attributable to smoking.

Of course, you also know that smoking-related diseases are usually preventable—and it is never too late to quit! Stopping smoking can give you health benefits right away. According to the American Cancer Society (ACS), within twenty minutes after you quit, your body starts regenerating and your blood pressure begins to return to normal. Within eight hours, the carbon monoxide level in your blood drops to normal. Twenty-four hours after you quit, your chance of heart attack begins to decrease. One to nine months later, you should lose that smoker's cough and the sinus congestion, fatigue, and shortness of breath smokers suffer. Within ten years of quitting, you will have cut your risk of lung-cancer death in half; after fifteen years, your chance of contracting coronary heart disease is the same as that of a nonsmoker.

 ## Fact

In 1999, the New England Journal of Medicine reported a study that found that nonsmokers exposed to environmental smoke have a higher risk of coronary heart disease than those who aren't. So don't be shy—ask smokers to smoke outside.

Smoking is an incredibly addictive habit that hooks you physically, psychologically, and emotionally. If you are struggling with quitting, talk to your doctor or health care provider about smoking cessation programs, nicotine replacement therapy, and other techniques that can help you kick the habit. If you have children, remind yourself of how important you are to them as a role model; your quitting smoking may help them decide not to start.

Controlling Your Risks

As you've probably determined by reading the previous sections on individual risk factors for developing heart disease, you actually can reduce your own risk for this disease and the conditions that contribute to it. Though you might have a genetic susceptibility to high blood pressure, high cholesterol, or diabetes, or your age itself may increase your chances of contracting heart disease, you can take positive action to manage your overall risks. Here are some suggestions:

- **Eat a low-fat, low-cholesterol, high-fiber diet.** The less saturated fat you consume, the better you'll be able to manage blood cholesterol levels. Try to build your diet around fresh fruits, vegetables, and whole grains. Limit the amount of animal fat, meat, and dairy products you consume, and go easy on the salt—especially if you suffer from high blood pressure.
- **Manage your weight.** Ask your health care provider to help you determine what your weight should be and how you can best reach and maintain that weight. No matter what other lifestyle changes you make, being overweight or obese can dramatically increase your risks of suffering from some form of heart disease.
- **Exercise regularly.** Physical activity not only helps control obesity, but also helps dramatically reduce the severity of many conditions that contribute to heart disease. The Surgeon General recommends thirty minutes of exercise, at least three days a week.
- **Drink alcohol in moderation.** If you drink alcohol, keep your consumption to no more than one drink a day.
- **Stop smoking.** Now—use whatever means necessary.
- **Find ways to avoid or relieve stress.** Being stressed out is not only unpleasant but also hard on your heart. When you're under stress, your heart rate can go up, your breathing can become shallow, and all of your muscles can become tense. If you want your heart and brain to be nourished by a strong, healthy flow of oxygenated blood, keep stress to a minimum. Exercise helps, as does relaxation therapy, meditation, and quiet time spent enjoying the things you love.

CHAPTER 15

Maintaining Bone Health

OSTEOPOROSIS IS A THREAT every woman should take seriously, and one that grows even more serious as menopause approaches. Your best defense against osteoporosis is to understand your risks for developing this disease and to follow a sensible plan for minimizing those risks and protecting your bones—for the rest of your life. This chapter will discuss what warning signs you should look out for and tips on how to change your lifestyle to promote healthy, strong bones.

Close-Up on Osteoporosis

Osteoporosis is a degenerative bone disease that every woman should view as a potential enemy. According to a 2004 Surgeon General's Report, by the year 2020 half of Americans over age fifty will be at risk of fracture and low bone mass. Ten million people already have osteoporosis, and another 34 million are at risk for developing it. What is really frightening is that 80 percent of the Americans either diagnosed or at heightened risk are women.

If your first instinct upon reading these statistics is to dash out and stock up on calcium supplements, hold on a minute. Your best weapon against osteoporosis is knowledge; take a moment to get the facts on this disease. Then, you can get the calcium supplements—and follow the simple prescription for bone health offered later in this chapter.

What Is Osteoporosis?

Osteoporosis is a disease in which your bones lose density. When you have osteoporosis, your bone tissue deteriorates, leaving your bones structurally weak and susceptible to fractures. Typically, victims of osteoporosis suffer fractures in their hips, spinal vertebrae, and wrists, but any bone in the body can crumble when this disease progresses to an advanced state.

Many people think of their adult bones the same way they view their home's framework: a stable and unchanging support for the growing, vital parts of the body's makeup. But bones are alive. Bone tissue is in a constant state of evolution, as the body replaces old bone cells with new bone cells. When you're a child, your bones have a lot of growing to do, so your body produces much more new bone than it takes back in through reabsorption (the process of absorbing old bone cells back into the body).

 # Fact

Fifty percent of women with osteoporosis don't have any recognizable risk factors, so all women should take precautions; eat a healthy, calcium-rich diet; get plenty of weight-bearing exercise; and get bone-density testing.

When Does It Happen?

Around age thirty-five, your body reaches a stage of peak bone mass, where your bones are as large and dense as they will ever be. At that stage, reabsorption slowly begins to outpace bone production. If reabsorption becomes too rapid or if bone cell production becomes too slow, you're at risk for developing osteoporosis. If you didn't build your bones to their optimum size during the years leading to peak bone mass, your risk is even greater.

Right now, there is no cure for osteoporosis. But you can slow the progress of the disease dramatically through a treatment plan involving some combination of medication, diet, and exercise. Recent experiments with drugs that may actually help rebuild lost bone tissue offer true encouragement to victims of this disease and those who treat them. But remember, prevention is easier than treatment.

Alert

Young girls need to build bone density, but it's not a subject that interests most teenagers. So, if you have a young daughter or niece, make sure she's taking an adequate amount of calcium, especially during her early teen years' growth spurt.

What to Watch For

Osteoporosis, even today, is under-diagnosed and under-treated. Like many deadly diseases, osteoporosis gains much of its power through its ability to progress silently without any apparent signs or symptoms. Bone tissue loss isn't painful in its early stages—everyone experiences it every day. Weak bones don't ache, or creak, or exhibit any other kind of warning. In fact, osteoporosis frequently is diagnosed only after someone suffers a bone fracture. And even then, if the person who suffered the break and/or her doctor doesn't suspect that the break could be related to osteoporosis, and follow up with the proper diagnostic tests, the disease can remain undiagnosed and untreated.

A Very Quiet, Very Large Problem

Osteoporotic bones lose mass very slowly; over time, the bones become so fragile that they can break under very slight strain. Every year, osteoporosis is responsible for:

- 300,000 hip fractures
- 700,000 vertebral fractures
- 250,000 wrist fractures
- 300,000 fractures at other sites

Some of these figures may be underestimates, since certain fractures aren't even recognized when they occur. The pain resulting from crumbled vertebrae might seem like a back strain, for example. If the broken bone goes unnoticed or, the break is apparent but no one connects it to the disease, osteoporosis continues to erode the bones until another fracture occurs. By the time the warning flag goes up, the disease may have advanced to a critical stage.

Essential

Ninety percent of all hip fractures are associated with osteoporosis and result from a fall. Most falls happen to women in their homes in the afternoon. As you get older and your legs lose strength, your eyesight weakens (especially your peripheral vision), and your balance and flexibility diminish, you're more likely to fall and less able to catch yourself.

Diagnosing the Disease

Because osteoporosis is such a well-hidden disease, your health care provider will turn to your health history (and your family's health history) to determine what your risk factors are for developing the disease. A close review of your osteoporosis risk profile will tell your health care provider how soon (and often) you need to be checked for the development of the disease.

The most common and effective diagnostic tool for osteoporosis is a bone-density measurement known as a bone mineral density (BMD) test. BMD tests can measure the density of the bones in your spine, wrist, heel, and/or hip.

The most common type of bone density test is a dual energy X-ray absorptiometry (DEXA) test. In this test, low-dose X-ray beams scan your lower (lumbar) spine and/or hips for ten to twenty minutes. The test isn't painful, and you're exposed to minimal radiation, so it's a safe and effective diagnostic tool. Other types of bone density scans use ultrasound to measure the bone mass in your heel or wrist, but aren't as conclusive as the DEXA test. However, a quick office scan of the density of your heel or wrist still provides very useful knowledge, especially if you are relatively young (less than forty-five years old), and have risk factors for this condition. This type of peripheral bone density testing is a great screening tool, because it takes fewer than two minutes to perform, and most doctors can conduct the test right in the office during a routine visit.

Besides warning you about osteoporosis before you suffer a fracture, bone-density tests can help you determine your rate of bone loss and help you gauge the effectiveness of your efforts to slow that loss. A BMD test can tell you how your bone density compares to that of healthy bone tissue from a person of your age and—more importantly—to that of an average thirty-year-old.

 Alert

Fractures from minor accidents can indicate bone loss. If you have suffered a fracture after a minor fall, you should ask your doctor about conducting a BMD test. Other late signs of osteoporosis occur in many women age sixty-five and older, including stooped shoulders or a loss of height.

Menopause and Osteoporosis

As you approach menopause, your chances for developing this disease increase dramatically. Here's why. Your bones are in a constant state of remodeling its bone tissue, by removing old bone tissue cells through reabsorption and creating new ones. But the body is more adept at tearing down the old than at building the new. Your body depends upon its growth hormones—especially estrogen—to help pace the remodeling process.

Estrogen Loss Depletes Bone Tissue

So what role does estrogen play in this whole remodeling process? Estrogen protects your bones by controlling the amount of bone removed by reabsorption. When your estrogen levels drop after menopause, your bones lose that protection. As a result, in the five to eight years following menopause, your bone loss can increase dramatically as your body adjusts to the loss of ovarian estrogen.

If you've gone through an early menopause, your body has endured a greater-than-normal estrogen loss and your risk of experiencing accelerated bone loss increases. And if you've ever experienced extensive or frequent bouts of amenorrhea (lack of periods), your bones have been through periods of accelerated bone loss due to a loss of estrogen protection.

 Fact

Your parathyroid gland secretes a hormone that controls the amount of calcium released by your bones into the bloodstream. If this gland becomes overactive (hyperparathyroidism), your bones can release too much calcium and contribute to the development of osteoporosis. This condition is particularly dangerous for women in menopause. The good news is that hyperparathyroidism is a treatable condition.

The Facts about Postmenopausal Bone Loss

Though your bone loss is gradual in the years between achieving peak bone mass and entering menopause, after menopause the loss increases dramatically. The average woman loses up to 3 percent of bone mass a year after menopause. According to the National Osteoporosis Foundation, women can lose up to 20 percent of their bone mass in just the first five to seven years following menopause.

So does that mean that every woman emerges from the first decade of menopause with thin, fragile bones? Certainly not! Remember that the condition of your bones plays a role in preserving their mass, as do a number of other factors, including heredity, environment, diet, and exercise.

All of these facts lead to only one logical conclusion: Every woman— regardless of her age or health—needs to understand her risks for developing osteoporosis and have a sound, ongoing plan for maintaining her bone health. Waiting until you're older or waiting until you've entered menopause to protect yourself against osteoporosis just won't work; by then, you could already be losing the battle against bone loss.

Understanding and Controlling Your Risks

If every woman goes through menopause, why doesn't every woman develop osteoporosis? The risk factors for developing this disease go well beyond age and hormonal production rates. As with heart disease and other midlife health risks, some are under your control and some are not. The trick is to be aware of all of them and focus on the ones that you can impact.

Common Risks for Bone Loss

There are some circumstances, traits, and habits that make women more likely to suffer from osteoporosis. Here are some of the genetic, environmental, and other risk factors for developing this disease:

- **Body makeup.** Women with thin, small frames are at greater risk of suffering excessive bone loss as they age.
- **A family history of osteoporosis.** If other women (or men) in your family developed this disease, your risk for developing it goes up.
- **Caucasian or Asian race.** African-American women have a much lower incidence of postmenopausal osteoporosis than do Northern European and Asian women. However, they still need the same screening for other risk factors.
- **Taking certain medications.** If you've taken steroids (such as prednisone), anticonvulsants, or lithium for more than three months, your risks for developing osteoporosis increase. If you are on thyroid replacement therapy, be sure the level is monitored, since taking too much can increase your risk for osteoporosis.
- **Eating disorders.** A history of eating disorders such as anorexia or bulimia can increase your risks. Infrequent or irregular periods can be a sign that excessive dieting is resulting in low estrogen levels.
- **Lifestyle choices.** Excess consumption of alcohol, inadequate calcium intake, cigarette smoking, and a lack of exercise all can contribute to the development of osteoporosis over time.

What You Can Do Right Now

As you can see, some risk factors are controllable and others aren't. But you have many options available to you for preventing or slowing the progress of osteoporosis. The National Osteoporosis Foundation recommends these four steps for preventing or managing the disease:

- Eat a healthy diet that includes ample supplies of calcium and vitamin D.
- Incorporate weight-bearing exercise, such as walking or weight-lifting, in your regular exercise plan (and that means doing these exercises three or more times a week).
- Stop smoking and don't overindulge in alcohol.
- If you're at high risk for osteoporosis, get a bone-density test. Your care provider can tell you when and how often it should be repeated.

 Fact

Osteoporosis-related fractures can be killers. In 2001, nearly 315,000 Americans age forty-five and older were hospitalized as a result of hip fractures, and osteoporosis was a contributor to most of these breaks. Mortality rises each decade, and by age eighty, 50 percent of patients who experience a hip fracture die within the year that follows their fracture.

Eating for Strong Bones

You already know that your diet plays a big role in your overall health, but a balanced diet rich in calcium and vitamin D is particularly important for preventing or slowing the progress of osteoporosis. Your body stores pounds of calcium in its bones, and calcium is an essential nutrient for all of your body's organs and tissues. Therefore, maintaining your calcium levels helps keep all of your body—not just its bones—healthy and fit.

A woman's calcium requirement changes as she ages. Between the ages of nine and eighteen, you should get at least 1,300 milligrams of calcium every day. You can drop that amount to 1,000 milligrams per day from ages nineteen to fifty. By the time you reach age fifty, you need at least 1,200 to 1,500 milligrams of calcium every day. (If you're still having periods or taking estrogen, the lower number will do, but if you're in menopause and not on estrogen, move up to the higher amount.) What foods give you the greatest calcium boost? Here are just some examples (remember to check food product labels):

Sources of Calcium	
Food	Milligrams of Calcium
Nonfat, plain yogurt, 1 cup	452
Swiss cheese, 1½ ounce	408
Macaroni and cheese, 1 cup	362
Sardines, canned with bones, 3 ounces	321
Skim milk, 1 cup	302
Whole milk, 1 cup	291
Tofu, 1 cup	260
Kale, cooked, 1 cup	179
Vanilla ice cream, 1 cup	170
Spinach, fresh or cooked, ½ cup	122
Almonds, ⅓ cup	114

But getting plenty of calcium isn't your only dietary weapon against osteoporosis. While vitamin D doesn't put more calcium into your system, it does help your body use the calcium you eat. Your body absorbs vitamin D from the sun; if you live in a cold or northern climate, or don't spend much time outdoors, vitamin D added to your calcium supplement will help your gastrointestinal system absorb the calcium. Women between the ages of fifty-one and seventy need about 800 units of vitamin D every day. You can get 25 percent of your daily requirement simply by drinking an eight-ounce glass of vitamin D-fortified milk every day. Eggs and some fish, including sardines, mackerel, and herring, contain small amounts of vitamin D.

Don't misunderstand: eating a well-balanced diet with adequate amounts of calcium and vitamin D won't guarantee an osteoporosis-free life. But without question it's the best method available for helping your body prevent or slow the disease.

 Question

Can you be a vegetarian and eat a bone-healthy diet?
Yes, you can! However, you must eat a well-balanced diet of beans, seeds, grains, and a broad variety of vegetables. Ovo-lacto vegetarians eat eggs and dairy products, and therefore have more access to calcium in their diet. If you eat no dairy products at all, you need to carefully monitor your calcium intake and consider supplements.

Using Calcium and Vitamin Supplements

Although diet is always the best source of vitamins and nutrients, as you approach menopause, you may find that your diet needs some boosters in the form of supplements. Some estimates indicate that most menopausal women eat only about half as much calcium as they require each day. And many women have trouble digesting dairy products, so upping their intake of milk, yogurt, and cheese may not be an option for getting the increased calcium their bones demand.

Calcium supplements are available in a number of forms today, and they can be a great benefit to any woman approaching menopause. Keep these facts in mind when choosing and using calcium supplements:

- The elemental calcium content of any supplement is what matters most. Check the label carefully to make sure the supplement carries the appropriate amount of elemental calcium.
- Choose calcium supplements from reputable makers; check the label to see if the calcium is purified and look for the USP

(United States Pharmacopoeia) symbol to help guarantee the reliability of the source.

- Calcium works best when you take it in 500 milligram doses, divided over the course of the day.

Because vitamin D is available in few nondairy foods, many people need to supplement their daily supply. Most all-purpose vitamins contain a daily dose of vitamin D, as do some calcium supplements. And minerals such as phosphorous and magnesium are important for bone health, too. Again, adequate doses of these are available in most multivitamins.

Remember, a well-balanced diet is always your best source of nutrients, including vitamins and minerals. But as women approach menopause, most find that they need supplements to round out their daily requirements of calcium. As with any health-related plan, however, discuss all dietary and food supplement decisions with your doctor or health care professional before making any changes in your current practices.

 Fact

Your body may be intolerant of a fast, sizeable increase of calcium; signs of that intolerance can be indigestion or gas. Try to build slowly toward your full dosage, and if your system continues to have problems, try a different calcium supplement. A calcium-supplemented orange juice may reduce these side effects.

Beyond Diet: Measures to Prevent Bone Loss

While diet and calcium intake are the foundation for maintaining bone density, they work in concert with other factors. Exercise, hormone therapy and medications all have their place in combating this disease. Your health care provider can discuss the options and combinations that would work best for you, depending on your risk profile and physical health.

Exercising as Prevention

You probably didn't hear it here first, but exercise is an absolute must for a healthy life—and a healthy passage through menopause. Exercise plays a particularly important role in protecting your bones. Studies have shown that weight-bearing exercise builds strong, healthy, resilient bones and can slow the progress of bone loss. Walking, one of the most popular forms of exercise, seems to be particularly helpful in encouraging new bone growth. Exercise not only helps maintain your bones' health but also keeps your joints and muscles flexible and strong. Those improvements alone go a long way toward helping you prevent fractures caused by falls.

Most health care professionals recommend thirty minutes of weight-bearing exercise—such as walking or other moderately intense physical activity—three days a week, as part of a total exercise program that also includes aerobic and stretching exercises. If you go with a weightlifting program, make sure you get the help and advice of your health care professional in planning a program that will offer you the maximum benefit and the minimum risk of strain or injury.

Exercise alone won't prevent osteoporosis. But if you combine a sensible exercise program with a well-balanced diet (remember those high levels of calcium and vitamin D) and avoid smoking and excess alcohol consumption, you'll go a long way to preserving your bone health, even after menopause.

 Fact

In addition to weight-bearing aerobic exercise, weight training (also called resistance training) can slow down the loss of bone and even increase bone mineral density. It also shows some evidence of improving balance, possibly from better muscle tone, thereby decreasing falls. Check with your health care provider, and then take a class in free weights. It could make all the difference!

Using Estrogen for Bone Health

Diet, exercise, and nutritional supplements can all slow the bone loss your body experiences after menopause, but they can't stop it. However, most doctors agree that estrogen therapy can halt bone loss during this time and may actually contribute to bone growth. Estrogen helps to activate the vitamin D in your body to enhance its ability to absorb calcium. It also promotes the production of collagen in your system that aids in the development of bone strength and flexibility.

Menopause hormone therapy (MHT) has been shown to reduce bone loss, increase bone density in the spine and hip, and reduce the risk of hip fractures in postmenopausal women. If you are approaching menopause, talk to your health care professional about the benefits and risks of estrogen for the prevention of osteoporosis after menopause. MHT is also beneficial for the eyes, colon, and joints, so try to discuss all these benefits with your physician.

 Alert

Some medications, such as corticosteroids, thyroid hormone replacement medications, and anticonvulsants, can contribute to bone loss. If your doctor prescribes these medications, be sure you have discussed your family health history and personal risks for osteoporosis.

Other Options for Slowing Bone Loss

If you are not a good candidate for MHT, and diet and exercise are not enough to keep your bones strong, you still have more options in the battle against bone loss. There are medications available that can slow the reabsorption of bones into your body, and are worth discussing with your health care provider.

Bisphosphonates

Bisphosphonates are anti-resorptive medications like alendronate (Fosomax) and risedronate (Actonel) used to slow down or block calcium loss from the bones. They are available in daily, weekly, or monthly dosages, and can be very effective in slowing bone loss. Other medications and supplements can interfere with their effectiveness, so it's best to take them in the morning before any other medications and with lots of water. They can have side effects such as irritation of the esophagus and osteonecrosis of the jaw, so discuss with your medical provider whether you would be a good candidate for these medications.

SERMs and "designer" estrogens

In addition to estrogen, some "designer" estrogens, including raloxifene and the bisphosphonates alendronate and risedronate have been approved by the Food and Drug Administration for the prevention and treatment of postmenopausal osteoporosis. Though these drugs don't share estrogen's other benefits, they may help to maintain bone density and represent a welcome alternative to estrogen for women who want a sound defense against osteoporosis, but who cannot or choose not to take estrogen in MHT (see Chapters 11 and 12 for a full discussion of HRT and its alternatives).

Fact

Calcitonin is the hormone your parathyroid gland produces to help control bone loss. The FDA has approved calcitonin, available in a prescription nasal spray, for treatment—not prevention—of osteoporosis.

Alendronate, risedronate, and raloxifene have been shown to reduce bone loss, increase bone density, and reduce the risk of fractures, just like estrogen. Raloxifene is among the newest of these designer estrogens, and it may offer some of the most attractive benefits. Raloxifene comes from a relatively new class of drugs called selective estrogen receptor modulators (SERMs) that prevent bone loss. According to the National Osteoporosis Foundation, early tests have shown that raloxifene increases bone mass and, after three years of use, can reduce the risk of spine fractures by about 50 percent.

Whether you choose to use natural estrogens, bisphosphonates, or designer estrogens to prevent postmenopausal bone loss, your doctor or health care professional is your best source of advice and information for making this important decision. But don't depend on either approach as your only solution for staving off bone loss. No matter what type of medications or supplements you take, a healthy diet and regular weight-bearing exercise are important components of your anti-osteoporosis arsenal.

- Alendronate is an FDA-approved bisphosphonate that helps slow the breakdown of bone tissue that occurs in osteoporosis. It is available in both daily and weekly dose formulations.
- Risedronate is a drug that inhibits the body's ability to reabsorb bone tissue, and thereby slows bone loss.
- Calcitonin is not really a nonhormonal treatment for osteoporosis but rather a hormone produced by the parathyroid gland and helps slow bone loss by slowing bone reabsorption, in a process similar to the previous two drugs in this list. It is offered as an injection or nasal spray.
- Raloxifene is an artificial hormone used as an alternative to estrogen. This medication has shown effectiveness in conserving bone mass, but does have a number of side effects, and is often a second choice to estrogen for women at high risk of osteoporosis.

Chapter 16

Eating for a Healthy Menopause

A healthy diet, supplemented with recommended vitamins and minerals, is your best tool for controlling or preventing some of the most damaging and debilitating conditions that affect women during and after menopause. The diet you've maintained from the age of twenty, however, is no longer adequate for the needs of your changing body. This chapter will discuss a woman's nutritional needs after forty and how to eat with both weight management and healthy living on the mind.

Your Nutritional Needs after Forty

A woman's body goes through significant changes during perimenopause; estrogen production slows dramatically, muscle mass decreases as fat deposits increase, metabolism slows down, body tissues—including those of the heart and circulatory system—lose elasticity, and the body begins reabsorbing bone cells at a faster rate than it produces them. For some women, stiff, aching joints; mood swings; feelings of lethargy; and insomnia join the list of physiological symptoms that accompany perimenopause. All of these symptoms contribute to serious health risks stemming from two oddly disparate yet closely linked conditions—overweight and undernourishment.

Good Nutrition Can Reduce Your Risk

The health risks of perimenopause and menopause include an increased risk of cardiovascular disease, diabetes, and osteoporosis. Add to these risks the health problems associated with overweight and obesity, and the challenges of maintaining your health as you approach menopause become painfully clear. Meeting these challenges requires a diet designed to both manage weight and boost nutrition.

What Should "Diet" Really Mean?

Many people go through life using their diets for everything but nutrition. They try one fad diet after another to lose weight; they load up on junk food and high-fat ice cream and chocolate as "food therapy" for overcoming anger, sadness, and disappointment; they choose foods based on convenience, portability, and easy cleanup. Though you may get by eating a shabby diet for a while, some time around your early forties, you may begin to feel the negative impact of bad eating habits. And even if you've always maintained a relatively healthy diet, you still may not be giving your changing body the nutrition it needs now.

What are the nutritional needs of women during and after menopause? Nutrition experts from the Institute of Medicine recommend these daily amounts of vitamins and minerals:

Recommended Daily Vitamins and Minerals

Nutrient (unit)	daily amount
Calcium (mg/d)	1,500 (1,200 with HRT)
Folate (mg/d)	400
Iodine (mg/d)	150
Iron (mg/d)	8
Magnesium (mg/d)	320
Niacin (mg/d)	14
Riboflavin (mg/d)	1.1
Selenium (mg/d)	55
Thiamine (mg/d)	1.1
Vitamin A (mg/d)	700
Vitamin B6 (mg/d)	1.5
Vitamin C (mg/d)	75
Vitamin D (mg/d)	10
Vitamin E (mg/d)	15
Zinc (mg/d)	8

Compiled by the National Policy and Resource Center on Nutrition and Aging, Florida International University, Rev. March 19, 2004

Question

> **Does it seem as if you're eating the same amount of food you've always eaten, yet you're gaining weight?**
> Your perception may be true; as women age, their metabolism slows down and they burn fewer calories in everything they do. So if your body is burning less energy while consuming the same amount of fuel, you will gain weight.

Nutritional Boosts for Women over Forty

Women approaching menopause have to pay special attention to the types and quantities of nutrients they consume each day. The following sections include just some of the special nutritional concerns for women at the age of menopause (remember that these amounts are general recommendations; women taking certain medications or combating specific conditions may need to take more or less, depending upon their doctor or health care professional's recommendations).

Vitamins and Minerals

While vitamins and minerals are always important to keep your body functioning, there are some that take center stage during menopause because changing hormone levels impact nutritional needs:

- Calcium is a woman's best friend as she approaches the age of menopause. Because the risk of developing osteoporosis increases as estrogen levels decrease, women need to be particularly careful to consume the recommended amount of calcium every day. If you're postmenopausal and taking HRT, you should consume 1,200 mg daily; if you're not taking HRT, and for all women sixty-five years of age or over, 1,500 mg is a must. Calcium is in milk, yogurt, cheese, and other dairy products, as well as in fortified fruit juices (see Chapter 15). Nevertheless, you may need to use supplements to get the full recommended amount.

- Vitamin D is an essential partner to the calcium in your diet. Vitamin D helps your body absorb and use calcium, and you can get 100 of the 800 IU (international units) recommended daily amount in one 8-ounce glass of skim milk. Some juices and certain brands of calcium supplements are also available with added vitamin D.

Fact

Although the FDA still recommends 800 IU as the daily requirement for vitamin D in women between fifty and seventy, research is showing that even women who get the recommended amount may be deficient. Many physicians are recommending a *minimum* of 800 IU of the vitamin every day to guard against low blood levels of vitamin D.

- Antioxidants, including vitamins A, C, E, and beta carotene, are vitamins found in a number of brightly colored fruits and vegetables. These are now considered important tools in warding off heart disease and some cancers, and may even reduce the deterioration of macular degeneration (age-related vision loss). Antioxidants work to stop the effects of oxidation within your body by protecting your body tissue from the effect of free radicals—molecules in your body that lack an electron and therefore "steal" one from other body cells. Like rust-proofing treatments for your car, antioxidants block these free radicals from damaging your body's tissues. Squash, sweet potatoes, spinach, mangos, tomatoes, red peppers, oranges, blueberries, and peaches are just some of the fresh fruit and vegetable sources of antioxidants. Chocolate may also provide some antioxidant benefits, but don't forget about calories when adding it to your diet.

Other Important Nutritional Elements

In addition to vitamins and minerals, your body needs other nutritional building blocks to meet your changing needs:

- Fiber is an important part of every woman's diet, and it's particularly important for women reaching the age of menopause. Women should eat 25 to 30 grams of fiber daily. Soluble fiber, found in fruit, vegetables, dried beans, barley, and oats, helps keep cholesterol levels low and can help prevent heart disease and lower the risk of stroke. Insoluble fiber, the type found in complex carbohydrates such as whole grains and the skins of fruits and vegetables, provides bulk that helps keep your digestive system on track and can help prevent colon cancer.

- Soy and other phytoestrogens can have a beneficial effect on your body as its natural hormone production slows down. Even though phytoestrogens are dramatically less potent than the body's natural estrogens, they can help alleviate some hormonal symptoms, such as hot flashes. Soy protein has real benefits for your heart; eating 25 mg daily can help lower LDL cholesterol by 5 to 10 percent. You find soy protein in soy milk (7 grams in 1 cup), veggie burger mix (11 grams in ½ cup), tofu (10 grams in 4 ounces), and roasted soy nuts (17 grams in ¼ cup), among other foods.

- Omega-3 fatty acids are found in fish, nuts, flaxseed, tofu, and soybean and canola oils. These essential fatty acids help nourish the hair, nails, and skin, but that isn't their only role in preserving health during menopause. New studies have shown that omega-3 fatty acids offer a number of benefits for cardiovascular health. The American Heart Association (AHA) reports that increasing the consumption of omega-3 fatty acids can benefit people who have pre-existing cardiovascular disease as well as those with healthy hearts and circulatory systems—especially when those fatty acids are consumed as part of a balanced diet. The AHA recommends two three-ounce servings of salmon, tuna, mackerel, herring, or other fatty fish every week. The FDA recommends no more than 3 grams per day of these essential fatty acids, with no more than 2 grams coming from supplements.

 Fact

According to the AHA, older Americans are less likely to die from cardiovascular disease if they eat at least two servings (6 ounces total cooked weight) of fatty fish every week. Research has shown that consuming omega-3 fatty acids reduces sudden death and arrhythmias, decreases risk of thrombosis (blood clot), lowers triglyceride levels, reduces growth of atherosclerotic plaque, improves arterial health, and lowers blood pressure.

Get It from Your Plate, Not a Pill

The best nutrition comes from food—not supplements. Though even a well-balanced diet might require the added benefit of vitamin and mineral supplements, those supplements should be used only to "top off" the nutrients supplied by food. If you aren't sure whether or not your current diet is giving you all of the nutrients you need, your doctor or health care professional can test your vitamin and mineral levels. Then, he or she can help you decide what (if any) supplements you need.

The Whole Is Greater Than the Sum of Its Nutrients

The American Dietetic Association (ADA) states that "wise food choices provide the necessary foundation for optimal nutrition." They point out that "many unidentified constituents that may have important health benefits are contained in the complex matrix of natural foods." In other words, you can't tell what you might be missing when you replace natural foods with supplements. So much is unknown about the interplay of nutrients that relying on supplements to ensure an adequate intake is probably unwise.

Alert

Don't forget the importance of drinking at least two to three quarts of water every day. Water is essential for cooling your body, transmitting nutrients throughout your system, and hydrating all of your body's tissues. When you're dieting and/or exercising, you must be especially careful to drink ample amounts of water throughout the day.

Food Is a "Package" Deal

Nutrients tend to be better absorbed from whole foods and may come in "nutrient bundles" that work together as they are absorbed. Because research is struggling to keep up with this area of study, it's hard to know what is lost when micronutrients are reduced to powders and pills, and whether the body can use them as effectively once they have been altered. A multivitamin mineral supplement is recommended, however, for anyone who is dieting, under stress, recovering from a recent illness, suffering from a chronic condition, or trying to boost his or her immune system.

Eating for Weight Management

Some changes that accompany age are linked to hormonal loss, while others appear to be linked to other natural processes of aging. Though medical science continues to study the causes and effects of the changes women experience in middle age, some facts remain clear and indisputable:

- As women age, they tend to lose muscle tissue and gain fat tissue.
- As women age, their metabolism slows down.
- As women age, their body fat is redistributed to their abdomen and midsection, unless they take estrogen replacement therapy, which helps maintain the traditional female fat distribution; in other words, keeping you looking pear shaped instead of apple shaped.

These facts don't mean that women are doomed to become fat and dumpy in middle age. However, as you consider how to construct a healthy diet for your midlife transition, you need to keep these realities in mind.

The Facts about Midlife Weight Gain

As your metabolism slows, you burn fewer calories; as your percentage of muscle tissue decreases and fat tissue increases, your body consumes fewer calories. These facts together mean that, all other things remaining equal, if you continue to consume the same number of calories through perimenopause and menopause that you consumed when you were premenopausal, you can expect to gain weight.

In one study conducted by the University of Pittsburgh, women gained an average of 2 kilograms (about 4.4 pounds) over three years of their menopausal transition. By eight years after menopause, the women gained an average of 5.5 kilograms (a little over 12 pounds). Though all women won't gain this much weight during menopause, many will—and some will gain even more. Without question, exercise is a must for controlling midlife weight gain (see Chapter 17). But eating a healthy, well-balanced diet is your other weapon to fight off this potentially deadly problem.

 Fact

To calculate how many calories you burn every day, multiply your weight by fifteen (if you're moderately active) or thirteen (if you get little exercise). The answer represents the approximate number of calories you burn during an average day.

Don't misunderstand the message here; a slight weight gain at midlife isn't necessarily a health risk. Women's bodies change during their transition, and the addition of one or two pounds is an expected part of that change. But overweight and obesity—as determined by a body mass index (BMI) of 25 or higher—are conditions associated with all sorts of health risks for men and women alike, including high cholesterol, high blood pressure, coronary heart disease, stroke, diabetes, osteoarthritis, and some cancers. The heavier you are, the harder you must work to move, and the less you feel like exercising. Being overweight can make you feel lethargic, depressed, and powerless—feelings no woman needs during her transition through menopause. There is some truth to the ironic observation that "the more you exercise, the more you feel like exercising; the less you exercise, the less you feel like exercising."

And the redistribution of body fat to your abdomen and midsection has dangerous implications. A large amount of abdominal fat is considered a high-risk factor for the development of diabetes and coronary heart disease.

Essential

Though slowing hormone production contributes to all of these (and many other) facts of life for most women over the age of forty, just beginning an HRT regimen without making any other adjustments is not going to solve all your problems. Make lifestyle changes—a healthy diet and ample exercise—part of any health management plan.

Temporary or Fad Diet Plans Aren't the Answer

Remember, when you read the word "diet" in this book, don't think about "the incredible all banana and cabbage weight-loss miracle" you read about on the Internet. Adopting and maintaining a healthy diet does not mean starving yourself or combining certain foods to magically block fat from being absorbed into your system. Long-term weight loss requires that you change your eating habits for good—not just until you drop that extra five or ten pounds. A healthy diet for long-term weight loss involves common sense: lowering your fat intake, lowering your simple sugar intake, and decreasing your portion size. In general, you must eliminate 3,500 calories from your system in order to lose a single pound of body fat. By lowering your calorie intake and increasing the number of calories you burn through a regular exercise program, you will lose weight. Stick to this program as a lifestyle change, and you will maintain a healthy weight.

 Alert

When you find yourself turning to food for the wrong reasons—to alleviate loneliness, boredom, fatigue, and so on—stop and think of something that will really help. Call a friend, take a short walk around the block, pick up a book, go to a movie, work in the garden, or write in a journal. Food won't solve any problem other than physical (not emotional or spiritual) hunger.

Good Eating Habits Aid Weight Control

A key component of managing weight gain during menopause is to develop good eating habits. Again, it really doesn't matter what's always worked for you before; your body is changing, and your eating patterns have to change, too, if you want to avoid excess weight gain. The following suggestions may help you:

- **Avoid fast food.** No matter how easy it is to grab a meal from the drive-through window or have it hustled to your door by a delivery person, fast food is packed with all of the things you don't need to eat, such as saturated fats, sugar, cholesterol, and salt. For the whopping 1,000 calories you may consume with that double bacon cheeseburger, you're getting precious little nourishment. Plan menus, shop for fresh produce, and learn to pack your lunch (with daytime snacks). If you have time on the weekend to prepare and bag fruit and vegetable salads, you can enjoy them through the week.

- **Try to enjoy your meals.** Sit down at a table whenever possible, and put your food on a plate rather than eating it out of your hand. Do not eat standing over the kitchen sink, and do not walk down the street eating a breakfast burrito. Take your time;

look at the food you're eating, smell it, and pay attention to each bite. Then, you're more likely to know when you're full. Shoveling food down while you stare at the television, drive to work, or read the paper by the kitchen sink is a sure ticket to overeating. If you really love to eat, do it with purpose.

- **Don't wait until you're starving to eat.** Try to eat small meals spaced out throughout the day. Eat a light breakfast, have a piece of fruit or a cup of yogurt midmorning, eat a healthy lunch, have a mid-afternoon snack, then enjoy a light dinner. The hungrier you are when you eat, the more likely you are to wolf down more food than you need. And the less cause you give your fat cells to get ready to sock it away. However, if you aren't hungry, don't eat. One of the biggest diet myths is that one absolutely has to have at least three meals a day. If you are not normally hungry in the morning, do not force yourself to eat breakfast.

- **Avoid eating late at night or right before going to bed.** Many people in the United States eat very little during the day, and then pack it away from the time they reach home until they go to bed at night—a very bad eating habit. You're active and at work during the day, so that's when you need your fuel. By the time you go to bed, your body should be ready to rest—not attempting to digest several pounds of recently consumed food.

- **Don't try to become a "food reformist" overnight.** If you need a dramatic diet makeover, take it in small steps. Give up one or two of your worst food habits at a time, and introduce healthy substitutes slowly. Start small—buy thin-sliced whole-wheat bread instead of white, try a new squash recipe, declare a weekly salad night, or skip the cookies and have a handful of grapes. If you don't want to completely turn your back on your favorite junk food, try limiting your quantities—maybe even set up a timeline, with a planned withdrawal period. Don't punish yourself about your eating habits—just work to make them better.

- **Keep a food journal for two weeks, where you write down everything you eat—including quantities!** It's essential that you know approximately how much you're eating. Many people think, "Oh, well, I had a spoonful of mashed potatoes, but that doesn't count." The fact is that everything you eat counts and your spoonful might be one-half cup, a cup, or more. That crisp green salad takes on some hefty calories when you ladle on the dressing; get out the tablespoon and measure how much you use (and check the label for calorie count). Weigh it, measure it, write it down. Then, you have a better idea of the amount of diet reformation you need.

- **Pay attention to portion sizes.** A protein serving should weigh about three ounces and be about the same size as a pack of cards. A serving of pasta is around one-half cup, not the plateful they bring you in most restaurants. One slice of bread or one cup of flaked cereal is one serving. A serving of fruit is one medium-sized fruit or one-half cup of fruit juice; vegetable serving sizes are one-half to one cup of raw or cooked vegetables.

 Alert

If you aren't accustomed to eating raw fruit and vegetables, add them gradually to your diet. These foods are essential to maintaining good health, but your system has to have time to adjust to digesting them. If you suddenly load your system up with an unusually high level of raw fruit and vegetables, you can have stomach pains, gas, and other gastrointestinal complaints.

Sane, Simple Guidelines for Healthy Eating

Putting together a healthy diet doesn't require that you have a Ph.D. in nutrition, a live-in cook, or a personal shopper. It just requires a little bit of education and a commitment to spend a little more time buying and preparing the right foods. This book isn't going to outline a week's worth of healthy meals; plenty of books do that already, and anyway, the choices are much too varied to be presented here.

There are some fundamental rules that can help you make sensible, healthy choices. Your daily food selections should include:

- At least three servings of whole grains
- At least three to six pieces of fruit a day
- At least two and a half cups of vegetables each day
- Two or three servings of protein foods such as fish, lean animal foods, beans, nuts, and seeds

Do's and Don'ts

As reminders for keeping your choices within a healthy range, here are some rules of thumb:

- **Limit your intake of fats;** total fat intake should be under 30 percent of all of your calories. Avoid trans fats and saturated fats. Fats in nuts, fatty fish, olive oil, flaxseed oil, and canola oil are healthier for you than are those in animal fats, shortening, and hydrogenated vegetable oils.
- **Eat a wide variety of fruit and vegetables of a variety of deep, rich colors.** Green leafy vegetables, oranges, tomatoes, squash, and blueberries are some of the low-fat, high-antioxidant foods you should include in your diet. Most produce sections carry a wide variety of vegetables and fruit, so why stick with the same old stuff you grew up eating? Try new things (by striving to eat foods the color of the rainbow, which will help you to expand your horizons and eat healthy foods you might otherwise skip), experiment, and focus on nutrition.
- **Limit your intake of salt;** high sodium levels contribute to high blood pressure, and too much salt actually inhibits the natural flavors of the food you eat. Taste your food before you add any salt. Also, consider a salt substitute, particularly if you are on a sodium-restricted diet.
- **Try to add "meno-healthy" foods into your diet.** Remember the benefits of fatty fishes—salmon, tuna, and so on—and eat some twice a week. Add soy to your diet, whether through soy milk, tofu, or roasted soy nut snacks. Don't dismiss these foods without trying them. They're high in nutrients and low in fat.
- **Be sensible about caffeine and alcohol consumption.** Caffeine has been shown to leach calcium from the body, and it can

aggravate conditions such as elevated blood pressure, anxiety, and tension. It's best if you limit your caffeine intake to just one or two servings a day, or consider switching from coffee to green tea—many green teas have only small quantities of caffeine and are rich in antioxidants. Don't drink more than one or two alcoholic beverages a day. Excess alcohol leads to a number of health problems, and alcohol is loaded with calories. Though most health experts agree that red wine has antioxidant qualities and can actually be good for you, keep your general consumption of alcohol low. You'll gain less weight and feel better.

Essential

Often, menopausal women feel that they're being forced to give up the foods they love as some sort of punishment for their age and sex. Your diet is one of the things you have complete control over, so be proud of your decision to eat the foods that will keep your body strong and healthy.

Your Own Revolution

The food you eat plays a major role in determining your long-term health. Maintaining a healthy diet doesn't require that you demonize every donut or treat each stack of pancakes as if it were a ticking time bomb. It simply means making thoughtful choices about the foods you eat and using food as a means to accomplish your health goals. Food is a great joy and an important part of many of our favorite family rituals—you should enjoy eating.

You'll never have a reason to regret improving your nutrition. No matter how many miraculous new medicines and treatments medical science develops for correcting the effects of disease or minimizing the changes that occur as we age, nothing will ever replace the health benefits of a well-balanced diet and regular exercise.

CHAPTER 17

Building Exercise into Your Menopause Plan

BY THE TIME they reach perimenopause, most women have developed some strong attitudes about exercise. Either you exercise regularly and can't imagine doing without it, or you've decided that exercise just isn't for you. Exercise is the perfect ally against many of the physical and emotional symptoms of perimenopause and menopause. This chapter explores the benefits of exercise for the menopausal woman and how to choose what exercises are best for you.

Why You Need Exercise Now

Sad but true: a woman's body is primed for weight gain in midlife. Although being unfit is never a good idea, it can seem particularly damaging after forty. Caught in a vicious circle of diminishing fitness, some women find themselves wanting to eat more and exercise less, just when their bodies need the opposite prescription!

The Midlife Slowdown

Even those women who maintain their same level of physical activity and food intake through menopause can expect to gain weight and lose muscle tone. This decline in fitness makes even a long-standing exercise program less effective than it used to be and more difficult to stick to. In the Healthy Women's Study conducted at the University of Pittsburgh, researchers found that by eight years after menopause, the women in their study gained an average of twelve pounds. The strongest predictor for that weight gain was decreased physical activity.

Does all of this mean that you're destined for fatness, not fitness, as you approach menopause? Absolutely not! These realities of midlife change simply mean that whatever your current fitness practices may be, they probably need an overhaul when you enter perimenopause.

If you've never followed an exercise program, if you've tried and abandoned regular exercise—even if you currently are following an exercise program that's been working for you over the past several years—you will need a new fitness plan as you go through menopause.

 Fact

According to the Surgeon General's Report on Physical Activity and Health, physical inactivity is more common among women than men. The report states that more than 60 percent of women in the United States get too little exercise, and 25 percent get no regular exercise at all.

Moving Less, Managing More

Your entry into midlife will undoubtedly be marked with some changes in your circumstances. If you allow life to slow you down at the same time you are taking on more and new responsibilities, your body will pay the price. Here's why you need exercise now:

- Your workday may be less physically demanding than at previous times in your life. At midlife, you may discover that you have become a "desk potato." Although you may feel as though you are constantly in motion, in reality you may only be going from sitting down to standing up more often, and not actually burning many calories.
- Your stress levels may be on the rise. As your career advances, the demands it places on you can increase accordingly. Economic and social upheavals, concerns over adolescent children and/or aging parents, and the onset of your own age-related aches and pains are just some of the stress makers you may face at midlife. Aside from its psychological toll, stress can cause chronic pain in your muscles, feed insomnia and fatigue, and trigger weight gain.

- After age fifty, your joint health and physical motor abilities can begin to deteriorate. As you lose balance and coordination, you become more likely to fall—and therefore less likely to participate in physical activities. Knees and hips can become stiff and painful, further damaging your interest or ability in leading a healthy, active life. Sadly, the less active you are, the faster (and further) these conditions develop.
- Your body shape and your body image may be changing at menopause. As your body takes on the natural contours of middle age, you may feel that you no longer have any control of your body's condition. Some women, feeling discouraged, may just want to give up. But throwing in the towel on fitness now can set the stage for a continuous decline in health, physical capability, and emotional well-being.

Essential

As you pass age forty, your risk of developing a number of life threatening age-related diseases begins to rise. Heart disease, diabetes, high blood pressure, elevated cholesterol levels, osteoporosis, and certain cancers are some of the serious conditions that menopausal women must guard against. Physical inactivity makes all of these conditions worse.

Exercise Can Save Your Life

A number of life-threatening diseases become greater health risks for women as they approach the age of menopause. While exercise is not the direct treatment for these diseases and conditions, it can be a valuable asset in their prevention and treatment.

An Excellent Tonic

Exercise has an impact on all of your body systems and supports body functioning as well as mental well-being. The combination is enough to make an enormous difference in helping your body combat all sorts of serious conditions. Here are just some of the potentially life-saving benefits of following a regular, sustained program of exercise:

- **Exercise makes your heart healthier.** Your heart is a muscle that grows weak with continued inactivity. The walls of an inactive woman's heart grow thin and are less effective at pumping blood throughout her system. Regular, aerobic exercise builds the heart along with other muscle tissues in the body. The walls of a physically active woman's heart grow thicker and stronger; her heart is healthier and does a better job of pumping nourishing blood throughout her circulatory system, especially under periods of physical or emotional stress.

- **Exercise helps keep cholesterol levels down and increases blood flow.** Even moderate levels of regular exercise can lower the level of LDL (so-called "bad") cholesterol in a woman's bloodstream. LDL cholesterol is responsible for the fatty deposits that collect on the walls of arteries, contributing to high blood pressure, heart attack, and stroke. A regular program of aerobic exercise contributes to clean, clear arteries that allow ample supplies of fresh, oxygenated blood to feed the heart and other body tissues.

- **Exercise helps prevent diabetes.** Diabetes is on the rise in the United States. The Centers for Disease Control and Prevention (CDC) estimate that 9 million women in the United States have been diagnosed with diabetes, and there are probably 3 million more who don't yet know they have it.

 Alert

Never begin any kind of exercise program without first discussing the details with your doctor or health care provider. Your health care professional can help assess your capacity for exercise and what type of exercise program might be the most beneficial for your particular needs.

- **Exercise builds strong bones.** Women who participate in little or no regular physical activity can lose at least 1 percent of their bone mass each year—even before menopause. Participating in regular weight-bearing exercise—including walking, running, climbing stairs, and dancing—can slow and even reverse this bone loss.
- **Exercise can help prevent some types of cancer.** Research from the American Cancer Society (ACS) reports that even moderate physical activity can lower breast cancer risk. Vigorous exercise has been linked to reduced risk for ovarian cancer and also reduces risks for developing colon cancer.
- **Exercise may help prevent or slow the development of Alzheimer's disease.** A 1998 study conducted by researchers at Case Western Reserve University School of Medicine and University Hospitals of Cleveland found that people who exercise regularly are less likely to develop Alzheimer's disease. Physically active people who do develop the disease are more likely to develop it late in life and experience a slower progression of symptoms.

Beyond the Body

Besides the effect on the brain itself, exercise improves mental well-being in general: Moderate exercise causes the brain to release more endorphins—naturally occurring substances that resemble opiates, and make you feel good and happy. The sense of satisfaction that you get from completing an exercise routine will carry over into the rest of your day, and may help with the discipline you need to stick to your healthy diet.

Managing Symptoms of Menopause

A healthy heart, strong bones, and a better chance for freedom from cancer, diabetes, heart disease, and other debilitating and fatal illnesses are all persuasive reasons to start exercising at any time of life. But menopausal women have even more to gain from following a program of regular, sustained exercise. Physical activity has been shown to help tame many of the menopausal symptoms that women hate most, including insomnia, hot flashes, anxiety, and mood swings.

Getting You Through the Change

Women who adopt a regular exercise routine notice that besides the preventive effect on the diseases that start to come in middle age, it can also help reduce or alleviate some of the most troublesome of their menopause symptoms as well. Here's a closer look at some of the meno-pause symptom-management benefits of exercise:

- **Exercise boosts your metabolism.** As you exercise, your metabo-lism speeds up, and it remains elevated for a while even after you stop exercising. The more energetic and sustained your exercise, the longer the metabolic boost lasts. An elevated metabolism helps your body burn more calories, which can help you lose weight.

- **Exercise may make you smarter.** In research conducted at Duke University and reported in the January 2001 issue of the *Journal of Aging and Physical Activity,* regular exercise was shown to improve significantly the cognitive functions of individuals over the age of fifty. In the study, participants who completed thirty minutes of aerobic exercise (walking, jogging, bicycling) three times a week experienced significant improvements in cogni-tive functions such as memory, planning, organization, and intellectual multitasking.

- **Exercise relieves depression.** In the same Duke University study, researchers also found that the relatively modest exercise pro-gram gave participants significant relief from the symptoms of major depression. After sixteen weeks, researchers found that those participants who practiced the regular exercise program had the same level of symptom relief as did those taking antide-pressant drugs.

- **Exercise helps you sleep.** Countless studies have shown that par-ticipating in a regular exercise program can help women go to sleep more quickly and experience fewer sleep interruptions. (Don't exercise right before going to bed, however; exercise leaves you feeling pumped up and can make it difficult to fall asleep right away.)

- **Exercise—both aerobic and strength training—has been shown to decrease hot flashes by as much as 55 percent.**
- **Exercise improves your endurance and makes you feel like moving.** Regular exercise strengthens muscles, builds endurance, and improves joint mobility and stability, enabling you to remain active and engaged in life.

Fitness as Menopause Therapy

Maintaining fitness is the most important component of your menopause management plan. Whether you intend to use hormone therapy or an alternative therapy, whether you have special risk factors for specific diseases or no personal or genetic-based risks, whether you experience all or none of the physical and emotional symptoms of perimenopause and menopause, staying fit is critical now and for the remaining years of your life. If you remain strong, active, and well nourished, you will experience fewer symptoms. You'll have greater resistance to any illness or disease, and you'll progress faster and more successfully through treatments for any condition that does develop.

But what does "fitness" mean? According to the American Physical Therapy Association, "a person who is physically fit has a properly aligned body structure; flexible and strong muscles; an efficient heart and healthy lungs; a good ratio of body fat to lean body mass; and good balance." Obviously, this will be different for every woman due to the vast differences in individuals' genetic makeup. Heredity also plays a role in how individuals respond to exercise. But your heavy parents or grandparents have not doomed you to being physically out of shape or unresponsive to exercise.

Fitness is based on the following six factors:

- Cardio-respiratory performance or aerobic endurance
- Muscular strength and endurance
- Flexibility
- Body composition—the amount of body fat and its distribution
- Bone density and strength
- Metabolic balance (how the body metabolizes glucose and insulin, blood lipid levels, and other metabolic actions)

L. Essential

> Because individual genetic makeup plays a major role in body fat composition and distribution, medical authorities carefully assess individuals when determining realistic goals for fat reduction. In addition to calculating BMI, your waist circumference and individual risk factors are all taken into account.

What Kind of Exercise Do You Need?

As unique as your individual fitness markers may be, a successful exercise program aims to improve three basic types of fitness: aerobic fitness, strength, and flexibility. The following sections take a closer look at each of these types of fitness with some examples of specific exercises for each.

Aerobic Fitness

Aerobic fitness is endurance fitness, or the prolonged ability to do activities requiring oxygen. Aerobic exercises make your heart work harder, speeding up your heart rate and sending more richly oxygenated blood coursing through your circulatory system to feed all of the tissues of your body. Aerobic exercise has many benefits:

- It builds strong, healthy heart muscle.
- It increases the capacity of your lungs, so you don't get short of breath.
- It helps your body regulate cholesterol levels and keep blood vessels clean and wide.
- It builds your muscle endurance and improves muscle strength.
- It burns calories and body fat.
- It builds resistance to disease, including diabetes, cancer, high blood pressure, and heart disease.

Remember that aerobic exercise is effective when it raises your resting heart rate—your normal heart rate during a period of inactivity—to a target heart rate, which is approximately 60 to 75 percent of your maximum heart rate. A treadmill or other fitness test can determine your maximum and target heart rates, but here is a general formula for finding a target heart rate:

1. Subtract your age from 220 to find an approximate maximum heart rate.
2. Multiply that number by 60 percent; the result is your low-end target heart rate.
3. Multiply the maximum heart rate number from step 1 by 75 percent; the result is your high-end target heart rate.

Any activity that gets your heart rate up and sustains it for fifteen to thirty minutes is an aerobic exercise; this category includes brisk walking, jogging, swimming, skiing, dancing, bicycling, rowing, hiking, rock climbing, stair climbing, cardio-boxing, and a host of other movement-related activities. The Centers for Disease Control and Prevention (CDC) recommend that adults participate in moderate-intensity aerobic activities for thirty minutes, three to five times a week.

 Fact

Aerobic exercises that include a weight-bearing component such as jogging, walking, step-training, dancing, and skiing build stronger bones and prevent the development of osteoporosis.

Studies have persistently shown that approximately half of people who begin an exercise program drop it within the first six months. If you want your commitment to exercise to last a lifetime, keep your interest up by changing and adapting it to match your growing fitness capabilities, interests, and needs.

L. Essential

There are many benefits of aerobic exercise, but they aren't permanent. To maintain aerobic fitness, you have to keep it up—try varying
the specific type, frequency, and intensity of aerobic exercise from
time to time. Your body needs continuous challenges to remain fit.

Strength Exercises

Weightlifting is not just for hulking bodybuilders. Now called strength
training or resistance training, it involves performing a series of repetitive, weight-bearing motions, usually using free weights or some other
means of providing resistance against the actions of your muscles.

Strength training improves your muscular strength and endurance, of course, but it also helps improve the health and mobility of
your joints. Strength training aids balance and coordination, and builds
strong bones—an especially important benefit for women in perimenopause or menopause. People of any age benefit from strength training;
many assisted living and convalescent centers incorporate strength-
training exercises in daily routines for even their bed- or wheelchair-
bound residents.

You have a number of options for incorporating strength-training
activities into your exercise program. Gym equipment such as most
Nautilus-type machines offer a great way to ease into resistance training. These machines have adjustable weight levels, and most help you
position your body properly to perform the exercises safely and get the
maximum benefit from your weightlifting action. A fitness instructor
can help you construct an exercise program that includes the use of
these machines.

You don't need to join a gym or buy expensive equipment to get a
good strength-training workout. You can buy a set of inexpensive free
weights to do arm curls and lifts at home. (You can even lift cans of soup
or full water bottles.) You can strap on arm and ankle weights while you
clean the house or take your daily walk. You can create a floor-work
exercise routine that incorporates traditional exercises such as sit-ups,

push-ups, leg lifts, and "air bicycling." Or you can buy a home-workout video that demonstrates any type of program that includes weight-bearing or resistance-training benefits.

In general, you perform weight-training exercises in sets of repetitions. Most people begin weightlifting, for example, with a weight they can lift six or eight times. You may begin by performing two or three sets of six or eight repetitions, and then gradually increase the number of repetitions and the amount of the weight over time. In general, people who want to lose weight but gain muscle tone should do more repetitions using less heavy weights; people who want to increase strength dramatically and bulk up should exercise with heavier weights but do fewer repetitions. Most medical and fitness experts agree that strength training should make up less of your total weekly fitness plan than your aerobic training.

 Alert

Be careful with yourself. If you have a fever or are recovering from a severe illness, don't push yourself to maintain your regular exercise routine; gradually return to your exercise program as you recover. Also, don't try to "work through the burn." If any exercise feels painful or exhausting, reduce the weight you're lifting, do fewer repetitions, or slow down.

Flexibility Training

Your flexibility is determined by the length, strength, and elasticity of your muscles and the range of motion of your joints. Joints require movement and use in order to remain flexible and functional. Long, inactive periods allow muscles and tendons to grow stiff; when that happens, your range of motion shrinks, and movements can become awkward and painful.

Flexibility is an important quality for any active life. Every time you need to stoop to pick up a child, turn around to lift something from the backseat of the car, or reach up to place canned goods on the top shelf of your cabinet, you call upon your ability to stretch your muscles and flex your joints. And flexibility contributes to good balance and coordination; if you slip on a wet floor or stumble over an obstacle in the dark, your flexibility may determine your ability to recover your balance and avoid a fall. If you do fall, you'll suffer less injury and recover more quickly if your body is flexible and strong.

 Essential

> Strength training is a powerful anti-aging strategy. It reduces the symptoms of many conditions including arthritis, diabetes, osteoporosis, obesity, back pain, and depression. You don't need expensive equipment or a trip to the gym. From push-ups to free weights, there are lots of ways to get started now!

Stretching is an important exercise for increasing flexibility. Remember, you should begin and end every exercise session with at least five minutes of stretching and warm-up movements. Flexibility training typically focuses on shoulders, hips, knees, and the hamstrings (muscles that extend up the back of your thighs). Stretches are slow, controlled movements that gently lengthen and tone the muscles and flex the joints, to give them increased elasticity and strength.

Fact

> Obesity contributes to osteoarthritis by putting an excessive load on weight-bearing joints (such as the hip and the knee). If you have this form of arthritis, however, your doctor will encourage you to exercise, both to help reduce your weight and rehabilitate damaged joints. A rehabilitation therapist can design an exercise program for your specific needs.

Choosing an Exercise Program

You have plenty of options for pulling together a sensible, effective exercise program that will give you the aerobic, strengthening, and flexibility training you need. The program you decide on should be fun for you; otherwise, you'll quickly lose interest. The following are some issues to consider:

- **Are you better suited to working out alone or are you motivated by working in a group?**
- **How much assistance will you need to begin your program?** You may prefer to begin with the on-site advice of a fitness instructor in a gym, and then do more of your work on your own.
- **Can you incorporate both indoor and outdoor exercises into your routine?** Designing an exercise plan that involves as much variety as possible is one way to make sure you'll remain interested and engaged in it.
- **How much money are you willing to spend on gym fees and equipment?** If you sign up for an expensive exercise program, the cost could become a reason to drop it after a short time. Look for seasonal price specials or introductory programs if price could become an issue for you.
- **Will the program you've chosen be convenient—or even doable—given your schedule?** If you choose a gym or workout center that's across town from your home and job, you'll be tempted to skip it more often. If you have to drag out heavy equipment or chase the rest of your family away from the television in order to work out, it may not take long before you decide it isn't worth the effort.
- **Does your program incorporate exercises that will help you build strength, aerobic endurance, and flexibility?** Don't create a program that's going to box you in to any one type of exercise or a single routine. By varying the type, intensity, and length of exercises within your program, you'll continue to challenge your body as its capabilities improve over time.

Helpful Workouts

Once you have decided exercise is your ticket through menopause, you have many ways to do it right. Talk about it with your health care provider, friends who exercise, and other people whose fitness level you admire. Ideally, you will choose an exercise routine that you enjoy and that offers you many rewards for your time. There are several exercise systems that offer a big payoff for the effort you put in.

Pilates

Pilates is a system of exercise developed by Joseph Pilates during and following World War I. A mixture of postures and movements based on ancient body practices, it stresses the importance of strengthening your "core" areas: your abdomen, back, and pelvic area, which are referred to as "the powerhouse." Using mat work and some special equipment, this program offers a combination of strength training and flexibility exercises, along with a mind/body focus and breathing techniques.

A regular Pilates workout can improve muscle strength, flexibility, posture, range of motion, circulation, coordination, balance, and mood.

Walking Programs

Walking is a simple way to get started in an exercise program. It is the perfect first step into a more active life. With a pair of comfortable walking shoes and a safe place to walk, you're in business. You can do it any time of year, and any time of day, so it is supremely adaptable to your busy life. A short daily lunch hour walk can get you started.

Once you are walking regularly, you could join a more formalized program if you want to increase the benefits. Many communities have walking programs on weekends, or "mall walking" opportunities in the early morning. There are group walks that you could explore, or you can find a walking buddy—human or canine—and hit the road several times a week. Walking briskly for a half hour three to five times a week offers many benefits, including stronger heart and lungs, better stamina, improved energy, and a feeling of well-being. What could be simpler?

Yoga and Tai Chi

Yoga is a term derived from a Sanskrit word meaning "union." It is a family of practices that lead to integration of body, mind, and spirit. Hatha yoga is the practice of assuming postures, called *asanas*, that build strength and flexibility. Like Pilates, yoga is practiced by people at all levels of fitness and focuses on bringing the body and mind together. Your body becomes stronger by holding the postures, your mind benefits from the concentration on doing the asana properly, and the breathing practices bring oxygen to your body, which refreshes and rejuvenates you.

Hatha yoga is a safe, gentle approach to becoming fit and the benefits include improvements in strength, flexibility, concentration, mood, and balance. Although breathing techniques are part of yoga practice, it is not usually performed as an aerobic activity, so combining it with a walking program is a well-balanced, adaptable approach to fitness.

Tai Chi is also an ancient practice with a growing following in the West. It is a Chinese traditional martial art combining slow precise movement with focused concentration and relaxed breathing to create a meditative yet physically challenging state. The *chi* refers to the body's energy, and Tai Chi helps you get that energy moving in ways that both invigorate and calm you. It is more meditative than yoga, but equally good for building strength, flexibility, coordination, circulation, and strength. It is perfect for the exercise beginner and, like yoga, can be done anywhere once the practices are learned. Yoga and Tai Chi have become staples of fitness in recent years. Their unassuming appearance might make them seem tame or uninteresting, but don't underestimate their powerful healing, conditioning, and stress reduction effects.

Exercise for Life

Finding the right workout or fitness program is a wonderful start for preparing you to meet menopause with open arms. Be open to suggestions and be creative. Hang around with your kids and play catch. Go for a long walk after dinner with a special friend or by yourself. Lift telephone books while you're on the phone. Put on your favorite dance music and hop around while you fold laundry. It's all about getting the blood moving again, any way you can. Every calorie you burn, every muscle you flex, every joint you move, gets you closer to your goal.

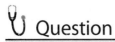

Question

I want a program I can commit to. What's a good way to start?
Walking has the lowest dropout rate of any exercise program. It's free, you don't need a lot of special equipment, and you can do it throughout your life. Most experts recommend walking more than three miles per hour if you are walking for weight loss. (You burn 416 calories per hour at that speed.) But don't forget to mix it up and add other activities to build a complete exercise program.

Don't give up! Even if you have to step away from your usual exercise routine for a few weeks due to work or illness, get back into it as soon as you can. Taking a positive step toward improving your physical condition is something to be proud of. Changes for the positive will be gradual, so don't be disappointed if the miracle transformation doesn't happen overnight. Keep at it, and you'll see the results.

Chapter 18

Keeping Your Mind Sharp

WITH PEOPLE LIVING LONGER than at any time in history, your surest chance for a happy and independent old age lies in keeping your mind finely tuned and functional for as long as you possibly can. Current research offers many ways to do exactly that. This chapter looks at steps you can take to keep you mind sharp and active.

How Your Brain Changes as You Age

Most medical and scientific authorities agree that the mind's ability to think clearly and quickly does change with age, but those changes aren't necessarily linked to menopause. Sometimes women mistake the transitory changes associated with hormone shifts for serious cognitive losses. It may be reassuring to note that the brain doesn't have a "use by" shelf life and that most nerves are capable of lasting 100 years or more. But changes in the brain's physical size and functions do occur with age, and those changes can have an impact on how well you access information stored in your brain.

Memory and the Frontal Lobes

The human brain shrinks slightly after age fifty as a result of a loss of water content. The shrinkage itself doesn't impair your memory, but the loss of frontal-lobe volume that accompanies that loss can. Some neuroscientists believe frontal lobes can shrink up to 30 percent between the ages of fifty and ninety. Frontal lobes are critical to complex thinking—your ability to reason, pay attention, and perform multiple tasks at the same time. A diminished capacity in your frontal lobes can diminish your abilities in all of these cognitive functions, and can interfere with some of your long-term memory functions.

Fact

> If you plan to live for a long time, you need to take good care of your mind. You can calculate how long you're likely to live online at *www.living to100.com* by taking Dr. Thomas Perls's "Living to 100 Life Expectancy Calculator," presented by the Alliance for Aging Research.

More Memory Functions in the Hippocampus

Perhaps most important to preserving memory and recall is the brain's hippocampus—the part of the brain where memory is created, stored, and retrieved. Some researchers believe the hippocampus can deteriorate with age—resulting in a slowdown of the brain's ability to store and retrieve memory. Exacerbating this slowdown are metabolic changes and a dwindling number of dendrites—the neurons that transmit the brain's signals. All of these changes can combine to affect your brain, making your mental sharpness feel duller and slower.

You don't need to panic that you're suffering an onset of early Alzheimer's disease every time you misplace your car keys—especially not as you approach the age of menopause. Many of the symptoms of menopause, including mood swings, sleeplessness, increased susceptibility to stress, and fluctuating levels of hormones, can contribute to less efficient cognitive functions—but most of these symptoms are relatively mild and transient.

Essential

> Not all the news about aging brains is bad. Studies show that myelination, the process of coating the brain with "white matter," continues throughout one's lifetime. This creates the capacity for more integrated and "big picture" thinking as a person ages, and can lead to the subtle developmental intelligence usually called "wisdom."

Give Your Brain the Nutrition It Needs

Your brain needs fuel in order to function. Some experts estimate that the brain uses 20 percent or more of the body's energy. Glucose and anti-oxidants are important components of your brain's nutrition, so make sure your diet includes plenty of whole grains, fruit, and vegetables.

Remember the Folates

The brain also may benefit from folates—found in leafy green vegetables, lentils, and other legumes. Folic acid, a laboratory produced version of folate, is included in many multivitamins and some fortified foods. Many studies also show that daily recommended doses of vitamin E and selenium may help slow the diminishment of cognitive functions. Recently, lipoic acid and coenzyme Q have been recognized to improve brain health, cognitive function, and memory.

What about Estrogen?

The research on whether estrogen preserves memory is not yet conclusive. The Women's Health Initiative (WHI) study showed that, contrary to anticipated results, estrogen therapy did not diminish or postpone dementia, and in fact women on estrogen therapy showed signs of dementia a bit earlier than those not on therapy. Although estrogen has been shown to improve neuropathways in the brain, not enough is known about how this happens to say that it definitely helps maintain your memory. Some studies suggest that it's actually the "enriched environment" of varied activities—both physical and cognitive—of women in the studies that makes the most difference in maintaining brain function, and not estrogen therapy per se.

Exercise Your Body to Keep Your Brain Healthy

The first step toward maintaining a healthy, active brain is to maintain a healthy, active body. Regular exercise—at least twenty minutes a day—is one great way to preserve your mental acuity. Aerobic exercise helps get the blood coursing through your system, carrying oxygen and glucose to your brain—two substances the brain needs in order to function.

Regular exercise also can prod the brain into producing more molecules that help protect and produce the brain's neurons. Though studies are still underway to establish the link between exercise and increased brain neurons, many researchers—including those involved with Alzheimer's disease research—are studying the protective effects of regular physical exercise on the brain's neural paths for transmitting signals.

 Fact

Physical exercise is a great way to reduce stress, and stress can take a serious toll on cognitive functions. Stress inhibits your ability to concentrate, and it can shorten your lifespan. The New England Centenarian Study has found that one trait common among those who live beyond the age of 100 is the ability to handle stress. (See Chapter 8 for other recommended stress-busters.)

Regulating Glucose

As you exercise, your body regulates glucose better. Losing weight, too, can help with glucose management. When glucose is properly regulated in your body, it protects the hippocampus, which in turn keeps your memory organizing ability intact. Research has used MRIs to show that people in better physical shape and whose glucose levels are within normal limits have larger hippocampuses and better memory function.

Exercise Your Brain to Keep It Lively

Some simple, but effective, techniques for putting your mind through some hoops to keep it active and highly functional are presented later in this chapter. But many of the most important things you can do to maintain your memory are really just good habits—things you do every day as a matter of course that keep your brain's neurons charged and firing and your hippocampus fully loaded and ready to dispense information.

What Cabbies and Musicians Have in Common

Mental exercise can increase the size of different areas of the brain, just as physical exercise increases muscle mass. Researchers have long known that musicians' brains are different as compared to those of non-musicians in that they develop unique patterns of brain activity from long hours of specific motor activities required when they practice. And a study of the brains of London cab drivers, reported in March 2000, indicated that specially developed capacities can continue into late adulthood. London cabbies are required to spend two years memorizing all of the streets, back alleys, shops, and businesses in London—information known as "The Knowledge"—then pass a memory test to get their licenses. Researchers found that the brain of a trained and licensed cabbie had a larger hippocampus than those found in the brains of a control group. And the hippocampus continued to enlarge as the cabbie used that knowledge. Cabbies who had been driving for some time—some for over forty years—had a larger hippocampus than their less-experienced colleagues.

Essential

When you're trying to memorize or recall something important, eliminate all other distractions. Turn off the television, lower the volume on the stereo, and get to a quiet place where people aren't chattering around you. You'll find you have to put in less time and effort if you are able to concentrate better, and you'll retain the information longer.

Good Habits to Keep You Thinking Clearly

You don't have to build a street map of London in your brain to improve your memory. But you do have to make some effort to "pump up" your memory. Here are a few tips to help you do just that:

- **Pay attention.** The first clue to preserving—or even improving—your memory is to learn to pay attention to what is being said and what is happening around you. Many researchers believe that inattentiveness is a major cause of forgetfulness in people of any age. If you don't learn to really listen and observe, your brain has no opportunity to absorb and store information. And pay attention to your actions as well; the classic lost-keys problem is easily resolved by creating a home-base spot where you always put your keys, for example. Write out lists of important things you must do, read the list out loud as you think about each item, and visualize some image or action that each represents to you.

- **Rehearse—slow down and repeat information.** When you hear a new name or have to commit a list of things to memory, stop, slow down, and repeat the information you have to remember several times. Repeat the name to yourself, and—if you've just met someone—repeat that person's name during the conversation, as in, "Well, Joanne, have you been living in the area long?" Rehearsing ideas and information aloud helps move information from your short term, working memory to your long-term memory.

- **Flex your brain muscles regularly.** Every day participate in some mental activity that requires your brain to remember, reason, and react quickly. Work a crossword or sudoku puzzle, play chess, draw, paint, or write in a journal.

Grabbing a few minutes of TV time may be a nice break from some intensive activity, but it's passive and doesn't challenge your brain to work on its own. Forcing your brain to learn something completely new is an excellent way to keep the neurons firing.

New Activities and Plenty of Rest: Recipe for a Sharp Mind

Learning new things, especially things that require new ways of thinking, or motor activities that you are not used to, is helpful in keeping brain tissue working. If you add a social component, it becomes more stimulating yet, and emotionally satisfying as well. Choose activities that lie within your areas of interest, and yet are novel and challenging.

Activities That Can Wake Up Your Brain Cells

To keep your brain cells flexible and expanding, consider one or more of these:

- Learn to play a musical instrument.
- Learn a new word game or study words for Scrabble, and then try them out.
- Join a group where you don't know any or many of the members.
- Change careers, or start a small business with your passion— for example, selling items on eBay or selling felted hats at craft fairs.
- Take up a new hobby that uses parts of your brain that you've neglected—for example, take a watercolors lesson or go kayaking on a calm lake.
- Learn a foreign language (and go somewhere where you can speak it!).

The more you exercise your brain's ability to think, the better it will function.

Get Enough Sleep to Keep Your Memory Strong

Research on sleep and memory reveals a critical relationship between the two. Sleep seems to help consolidate memories acquired during the day. Interestingly, the memory process appears to be more vulnerable at some times than others. And information learned during the day may be "lost" temporarily and then recalled after a good night's sleep. Scientists are still trying to sort out the details of this process, but it is becoming increasingly clear that sleeping well enhances your ability to remember and perform.

Another finding in the sleep and memory research shows that people with chronic sleep deprivation show signs of early changes usually associated with aging. Not only does a lack of sleep diminish memory, it also produces changes in endocrine function and glucose tolerance and is thought to hasten and worsen such age-related conditions as hypertension, diabetes, and obesity.

Most doctors agree that keeping your memory alive and well is a matter of following the basic advice offered throughout this section of the chapter: eat right, exercise your body, get enough sleep, and exercise your mind. But you can also use a few memory enhancing quizzes, games, and techniques to build your total recall.

Alert

Watch out for alcohol and other mind-numbing drugs. Most experts agree that a drink a day isn't health threatening, but drinking too much can deaden your brain's ability to retain and recall information. Abuse of alcohol or recreational drugs can result in a limited ability to form new memories.

Methods to Enhance Your Memory

Though most doctors agree that you don't need any formal mental gymnastics to keep your brain fit and functioning, many people have found that certain techniques or activities have helped them sharpen their memory. The simple techniques offered here can give you a leg up in bolstering your ability to learn and recall new information.

Tips for Capturing Information

Imagine this scenario: You're getting ready for work in the morning, and one of those morning news television programs is chattering away in the background. You hear one of the announcers mention a product development that gives you an idea for one of the projects your team is involved in at work. You tell yourself you're going to research the product further once you hit the office and discuss your ideas with your team. But by the time you're backing your car out of the driveway, you've put the whole thing out of your mind. When you get to work, you have a sense that there's something you were going to do, but . . .

Events, ideas, information that pass into the hippocampus will pass right on out again—unless you do something to lock them down by associating them with other memory that is already safely stored and ready for retrieval. The more associations the memory is tied to, the more likely you are to be able to store and retrieve it later. In psychology, this technique of associating new information with a range of memories for stronger recall is called elaborative encoding. It takes place in your frontal lobes—an area of your brain that always can use a good workout. Over time, people have used a number of memory devices to aid this process:

- **Use the "Roman Room."** Ancient Romans used this practice to help them memorize long speeches, lists of objects, city names, and so on. To try it, envision a room. Then place around the room visual cues that remind you of items from your to-do list, shopping list, or other types of information. A coat draped over a chair reminds you of the dry cleaning. A pair of skis leaning in the corner reminds you to call the travel agent about your winter vacation. Travel around the room in your mind, and make a mental note of sensory cues given off by the items—the colors, sounds, and smells of the items, how they coexist with each other, and any reaction they evoke in you. Make the images as vivid and compelling as possible. The room should exist in your mind as a real place, with each of its furnishings a reminder of the things, people, or events you want to lock in your memory.

- **Group or "chunk" ideas and information.** If you break down information into manageable "chunks" it is easier to remember. For example, a phone number, such as 1234567, is easier to remember when hyphenated: 123-4567.

- **Cue Yourself.** If you are driving and want to remember to run an errand or call the plumber, think of something that represents that task with something unavoidable. Think of pulling into the driveway and seeing a mailbox in the way (mail that letter). Or picture the toilet sitting in the middle of your front porch (call the plumber). These visual associations can help you hang onto your thought until you can do it or write it down. Another cue can be a verbal cue, like the ones we use to remember common things ("I before E except after C" or "Righty Tighty, Lefty Loosey" for which direction tightens or loosens caps, screws, etc.)

- **PQRST.** For complicated tasks like learning how to add numbers to your cell phone or using voicemail in a new job, you can follow these five steps: Preview, or skim the text of the instruction manual. Develop Questions that sum up the main points you need to learn. Reread the information again to answer these questions. Study the answers until you understand them. Test yourself by trying out the process—enter some numbers into your phone, or leave yourself messages on voicemail and then retrieve them.

- **Go into training for long-term lockdown.** When you have stored information in your long-term memory—not just until you leave work or get through tomorrow's meeting—put your memory technique into a training program. Review the information you need to remember at least three times a day for the next three to five days. At the end of your training program, you should have the information safely in the vault.

Organization Can Help Too

Maybe you are pretty good at making lists and using other tricks for grabbing that idea as it darts through your mind, but you need to set up a bit of structure to make that job easier. Here are a couple of organizational suggestions that may help:

- **Use external aids.** Keep tools around that make jogging your memory easy. Writing pads, lists of emergency numbers, appointment books, a personal digital assistant (PDA) with all your information in one place, timers, and an "outbox" to put things that remind you of outside errands. If you need to "take notes" in places like the car or the bus, many cell phones, PDAs, and MP3 players have a digital recorder on which you can dictate thoughts for later.
- **Organize the environment.** Arrange items in your environment to help you remember common things—for example, hang your keys on a hook just inside the door and put your medication next to your toothbrush where you can't miss it in the morning.

Most of all, work hard at preserving and building your cognitive functions, but try to enjoy the ride. After all, if you're worried about your memory, you probably aren't too far down the forgetfulness trail to get your ability to store and recall new information back up to speed.

CHAPTER 19

Taking Care of All of You

THE PHYSICAL AND emotional changes that come with menopause may put demands on your body and mind that you've never experienced before. Paying extra attention to a few body care basics can help minimize the effects of aging and keep you feeling fit and refreshed through your busy days and nights.

Appreciating the Woman in the Mirror

As you read about menopause and the special health concerns that accompany the aging process, you might start to feel like your body is simply a collection of potential problems. While it's true that the human body becomes more susceptible to certain conditions with age, you are much more than body parts in need of attention. You're a woman, with a life full of interests, and disease prevention may be a distant priority on your list.

Be a Role Model, Not a Fashion Model

Every woman expects the natural changes of age to occur, but in a culture that seems to worship eternal youth, rail-like thinness, and non-stop sexual vigor and allure, maintaining an appreciation and respect for your body as it ages can be difficult. One of the benefits of maturity is a growing appreciation for the valuable things that popular culture often fails to acknowledge. If you continue to compare yourself to every twenty-year-old you know, you are signing up for disappointment.

You can be a role model for all the younger women in your life. By accepting yourself and valuing humor, maturity, compassion, and other qualities over looking like a mannequin, you help redefine what it is to be a woman. Most women do *not* look like the airbrushed photos in the magazines, so finding a way to be comfortable with "normal" is a gift to all the women you know.

 Fact

According to the National Center for Health Statistics, the average woman in the United States over the age of twenty is just under 5'4" tall and weighs 164 pounds. Some studies of women in the fashion industry reveal that the average fashion model is 5'11" tall and weighs 117 pounds. You can see for yourself how far the reality is from the "ideal."

Start with Who You Are Today

The surest way to look your best is to acknowledge and appreciate the woman you are right now. Focus your attention on keeping that woman as healthy and happy as you possibly can. If you feel better, you will look better. Eat the foods that are right for you, follow the exercise program you need, keep every one of your annual health-maintenance checkups, give your skin and hair the extra care they need, and pamper yourself with the extra rest and relaxation you deserve. Taking good care of the woman you are today is the first and most important secret to looking and feeling your best through menopause and beyond.

Changes in Vision

Your reality and perceptions are formed by the information you take in through your senses, anything you can do to keep your sensory organs in top running order will make your life more comfortable and effective.

What Changes Will Occur?

Though few women need to worry about quickly losing their vision as they near the age of menopause, it can begin to diminish around the age of forty or fifty. We live in a visual culture, and most women agree that a high quality of life depends on their ability to see. There are a number of ways to protect this very important faculty.

Essential

Some medications can change your vision, either by reducing your ability to focus or by reducing your eyes' lubrication, making them dry and itchy. If you notice changes in your vision shortly after you've begun taking a new medication, contact the doctor who prescribed the medication and report the change immediately.

Monitoring Changes in Vision

Around the age of forty, many women begin to experience changes in vision. The shape of your eyeball can change as you age, and the subsequent reduction of your visual acuity can be subtle at first. Here are a few of the most common problems you might encounter after age forty:

- You may develop problems reading small print or seeing objects clearly that are close to your eyes. This condition is known as presbyopia, and usually is easy to correct with reading glasses, or even over-the-counter magnifying glasses from the drugstore.
- You might begin to notice tiny specks or odd dust-like particles passing before your vision. These "floaters" usually are just a normal condition of the aging eye. If they become extreme in number, or are accompanied by bright flashes of light, you should contact your ophthalmologist immediately. A sudden increase in the numbers of floaters can be a warning of a retinal tear or other more serious vision problem.
- You may experience problems with your eyes becoming dry and irritated after you spend some time reading or working at the computer. Again, this problem isn't unusual in over-forty eyes, and you may be able to alleviate it by using "artificial tears" (available over the counter in most drugstores) for better lubrication.

Alert

> If you work at a computer, don't allow your eyes to focus for long periods of time on the screen. Follow the 20/20/20 rule: Every 20 minutes look up from the computer at something 20 feet away for at least 20 seconds. Overuse and strain can take a toll on eyes, and long, uninterrupted hours at the computer can contribute to the damage.

Vision Problems to Watch For

Some people experience a substantial loss in the quality of their vision before they realize that the problem even exists. That's why all women (and men for that matter) after the age of forty should get regular annual eye examinations by an ophthalmologist. Women over the age of fifty are at particular risk of developing eye diseases, some of which might be connected to the loss of the body's natural estrogens. Your ophthalmologist will check for the following age-related diseases during your exam.

Macular Degeneration

Macular degeneration attacks the center of the retina, so central vision diminishes while peripheral vision remains unchanged. Macular degeneration can make reading and driving impossible; it's the number one cause of blindness in women age sixty-five and over. Its risk factors include being menopausal or postmenopausal, a family history of the disease, smoking, perhaps high blood pressure, and overexposure to the sun and other ultraviolet (UV) rays.

Although there is not yet a cure for macular degeneration, there are treatments that can stop the progression in some people. Prevention of the damage is the best course, and high intake of green, leafy vegetables has been shown to slow the progression of the disease.

There are studies that suggest that estrogen replacement helps postpone or prevent the onset of macular degeneration. The National Eye Institute conducted a study on age-related eye disease that showed a 25 percent reduction in the risk of developing age-related macular degeneration when taking antioxidants and zinc in these dosages: 400 IU of vitamin E, 500 mg of vitamin C, 25,000 IU of vitamin A, 80 mg of zinc, and 2 mg of copper. You can't get these dosages even in a well-balanced diet, so if you have a high risk of age-related macular degeneration, consider taking this combination to stave off the disease; talk to your doctor for more information.

Glaucoma

Glaucoma damages the optic nerve and is caused by a buildup of fluid, and thus pressure, inside the eye. When doctors detect and treat glaucoma early, the eye can escape permanent nerve damage. Chronic glaucoma develops slowly and, in most cases, is only detectable in its early stage through an eye examination. Acute glaucoma can happen suddenly, blurring the vision and causing a number of symptoms including nausea and dizziness. Risk factors include being over forty, being African American, having a family history of glaucoma, having diabetes, or being nearsighted.

 Fact

Doctors can't reverse the optic nerve damage caused by glaucoma, so early detection is essential. Ophthalmologists can test for glaucoma using a number of procedures. The simplest of these tests involves applying a short burst of air to your eye and determining how the surface of the eye responds to the pressure.

Cataracts

Cataract (clouding of the eye lens) risk increases with age. Some common symptoms include cloudy or blurry vision, fading color vision, "halos" around lights, or poor night vision. Your risk is higher if you have diabetes, spend long periods in bright daylight, or use tobacco or alcohol. In early stages, it is sometimes treated with prescription lenses, better lighting, or magnifying lenses. But if the lens is badly clouded, surgery removing the lens and replacing it with an artificial lens may be necessary.

Don't Be Shortsighted about Your Vision!

Your best prescription for maintaining good eye health after age forty includes:

- Getting regular annual eye examinations by an ophthalmologist
- Eating a healthy diet, including your full daily nutritional requirements
- Noticing and reporting to your doctor or ophthalmologist vision changes such as reduced night vision, clouded or blurry vision, bright flashes in your peripheral vision, or changes in your perception of color
- Wearing good UV-resistant eye protection while outdoors

Protecting Your Hearing

After age fifty, many women experience some hearing loss, and by age sixty-five nearly one-third of all women have some decline in hearing. You might not be aware that your hearing is fading until someone you live or work with brings it to your attention. Most age-related hearing loss is gradual and can develop slowly over a period of years.

Types of Hearing Loss

Some types of hearing loss can be the result of a physical injury, an infection, medication, or the development of growths or tumors. These hearing losses are called sensorineural (caused by damage to the nerves that transmit sound from the ear to the brain), because the sensors in the inner ear lose their ability to send sound signals to the brain. Long-term exposure to loud noise causes this type of hearing loss, so if you spent the 1960s with your ears glued to the loud speakers at rock concerts, you could experience this type of hearing loss.

Conductive hearing loss occurs when sounds don't reach your inner ear properly due to problems with something other than the transmitting nerves themselves. If you have a history of ear infections, damage to your eardrum, or even accumulations of earwax within your ear canal, you can experience this type of hearing loss. And, as the tissue within the ear canal becomes thinner and drier, it becomes less effective at transmitting sound.

⊑. Essential

Working near loud machinery, including lawn mowers and leaf blowers, can cause serious harm to your hearing. Avoid loud noise when you can. When you can't avoid the noise, wear earplugs or protective headphones. You may feel like an old-timer when you move to the back of the concert crowd, but there's nothing young and sexy about losing your hearing.

Keep Your Ear to the Ground

Regular hearing checkups can reveal either type of hearing damage, but you also need to pay attention to changes in your hearing. If you notice that you're turning the television up louder these days or constantly asking people to repeat what they've just said to you, you're probably experiencing some hearing damage. Losing your hearing can make you feel isolated and out of touch with the world around you. Take steps to protect your ears and monitor changes so that you can correct developing problems before they become irreversible.

Keeping Teeth Healthy

You know about the importance of regular dental checkups, brushing, and flossing. But did you know that menopause can present some special challenges to your dental health? As your body's natural estrogen supply diminishes in menopause, your gum tissues can become thinner and less elastic, and bone loss can contribute to the development of gingivitis and periodontitis—gum diseases in which the soft tissue of the jaw deteriorates around the roots of the teeth.

Loose Teeth May Be a Warning

If the bone density of the jaw itself diminishes, the socket of the tooth loosens its grip, and tooth loss can result. Osteoporosis in the rest of the body can be a silent process, but greater numbers of dentists are noticing loose teeth in their menopausal patients as the first overt sign of decreasing bone density in the body overall.

 ## Alert

> Gum disease is not just about losing your teeth. There is evidence that periodontal disease is actually a risk factor for coronary heart disease and stroke. Ongoing inflammation of gum tissue can introduce infection to the blood stream, where it can migrate to other organs and cause disease. Good dental hygiene and daily flossing can help you reduce this risk.

Make It a Habit

Some estimates show that over one-third of all women over the age of sixty have lost most or all of their teeth. To avoid joining that group, here's a simple plan for maintaining your dental health after forty:

- See your dentist twice a year for checkups and cleaning.
- Brush your teeth at least twice a day; use a soft toothbrush and floss afterward. Brush for two to five minutes, morning and evening (a third cleaning after lunch would be even better)—according to the Chicago Dental Society, it takes at least two minutes of brushing to remove plaque and bacteria.
- Make sure you're getting enough calcium in your diet, and limit the amount of sugar you consume.
- Pay special attention to signs of gum disease, such as bleeding or inflamed gums.
- Drink plenty of water—thirty-two to sixty-four ounces every day. Water can help rinse bacteria from your gum tissue and keep the tissue moist and healthy.

L, Essential

Those "water spray" tooth cleaners aren't as effective as a soft-bristle toothbrush and dental floss at removing tartar and plaque buildup between teeth—the number one cause of gingivitis. Plaque-removing mouthwashes can help soften and loosen plaque. Take the time to clean your teeth right to avoid the pain (and potential tooth loss) of gum disease.

If you have the time to floss only once a day, do it at night, right before you go to sleep. That's also a good time to use anti-plaque or fluoride rinses; you'll have a six- to eight-hour period without eating or drinking, so you can absorb protective fluoride and antibacterial agents.

Caring for Your Skin and Hair

If you have had no other signs of the passing years, you're likely to see some changes reflected in your hair and skin. As skin ages it loses elasticity and becomes thinner, drier, and more prone to itching and sagging. Your hair becomes thinner, too; it breaks more easily and grows in more slowly. Some of these changes are due to the body's diminishing levels of estrogen. Estrogen helps keep healthy tissues well nourished and moisturized; without it, both skin and hair lose strength and elasticity and grow thinner. Other changes are the result of age; as you grow older, your body slows in its production of new cells, and collagen production slows. Collagen is the basic bridgework, or support system, for all the fibrous tissue of your body, of which skin is only one component. Normal collagen helps keep the skin plump and resilient, providing part of the skin's support structure. Taking estrogen helps maintain the proper collagen content in tissues throughout your body.

Fact

> It has long been thought that waning estrogen accounts for the higher rate of age-related hearing loss in women. Studies, however, have not shown an improvement in hearing with menopause hormone therapy. In fact, studies show hearing loss associated when the artificial progesterone progestin is used in hormone therapy. If you are taking combination hormone therapy and have noticed some hearing loss, talk to your health care provider.

Exposure to the sun is another culprit in the deterioration of your skin's elasticity and moisture. The ultraviolet (UV) rays of the sun begin damaging the skin of young children; as sun exposure builds over the years, the damage becomes increasingly severe and apparent. Proper use of sunscreen with enough UV protection (SPF 15 or higher) and using hats or caps and sunglasses to shade your face and eyes may delay or prevent this damage.

Skin Care Basics

Your diet, the amount of rest you get every day, the level of stress you're subjected to, and the types of pollutants that exist in your environment all play a role in the health and vitality of your skin. Women in the United States spend millions of dollars every year on skin-rejuvenating treatments, including:

- Chemical peels and dermabrasion treatments that remove the outer layers of the skin
- Injections of botulinum toxin (botox) that temporarily paralyze the facial muscles to eliminate frown lines and other wrinkles in the face and neck
- Collagen injections that temporarily plump up the skin's understructure

- Radiofrequency treatments to the underlying collagen that tighten structures and stimulate collagen production, without surgery or injections.
- Cosmetic surgery that tightens, tucks, and lifts skin to eliminate wrinkling and sagging

All of these treatment options can improve the appearance of aging skin, but some of those improvements are expensive and temporary. And—as with any medical treatment—all of these techniques carry some risks, which, though infrequent, include scarring and skin discoloration. Carefully research any treatment option you're considering by getting multiple professional opinions and by talking to others who have used the procedure.

Essential

The fluctuations in hormone levels you experience during perimenopause and menopause can result in a relative increase in androgen levels as compared to estrogen levels. As androgen levels rise, facial hairs can become thicker, darker, more numerous, and more noticeable. Rogue chin hairs are a common occurrence for women age forty and over.

If you prefer to pursue less invasive techniques for keeping your skin looking healthy and vital, you have many options to choose from. Though your skin is unique, most women need to moisturize their skin more frequently after age forty. A number of creams, lotions, and even some prescription drugs are available today for nourishing and healing aging skin:

- Creams and lotions containing alpha hydroxy acids (AHAs) dissolve the upper layer of skin that has suffered the most damage to reveal fresher, plumper skin beneath. These products won't eliminate deep wrinkles or age spots, but they can make the skin look and feel fresher. Women with sensitive skin or rosacea should not use these products without the advice of a health care professional.

- Oils, creams, and lotions containing antioxidants and vitamin derivatives may help protect collagen, moisturize the skin's upper layer, and help diminish the visible signs of fine wrinkles. Vitamins C, E, and A are typical antioxidants used in these products.
- Retinol, a vitamin A derivative, is also a common anti-aging formula component. Prescription drugs Retin-A and Renova are marketed to reduce fine-line wrinkles, build collagen, and help fade age spots.

 Fact

Don't rely on magazine articles, a facialist, or a cosmetic salesperson for skin care advice. Talk to a plastic surgeon or a dermatologist about your skin concerns. He or she can help you pinpoint specific skin problems you might be developing and tell you the best techniques for combating them.

Beyond skin care formulas, however, you have some very basic tools at your disposal for protecting your skin. No matter what other skin care treatments you use, follow these basic practices to protect your skin and keep it looking its best:

- Drink at least thirty-two ounces of water every day—sixty-four ounces is better.
- Stop smoking—smoking ages the skin, breaks down its collagen structure, and increases wrinkles and sagging, especially around the mouth and the eyes.
- Anytime you go outdoors, use a sunscreen with an SPF of 15 or higher, even if skies are overcast.

- Maintain a daily skin care routine of gentle washing in luke-warm water, using a very mild soap. Avoid soaps with excessive perfumes and deodorizing chemicals, and don't scrub your skin!
- Use a moisturizer everywhere your skin feels dry, but especially around your eyes, mouth, throat, and hands.

Keeping Your Hair Healthy and Strong

The changes in your hair growth and health in perimenopause and postmenopause can seem downright unfair; the hair on your scalp starts to become thin, sparse, and gray, while some of the previously fine, pale hairs on your face grow thicker and darker. You can tweeze, wax, chemically dissolve unwanted facial hair, or use electrolysis or laser treatment to destroy the hair follicle permanently. (Some women experience skin irritation from laser and electrolysis.) Though some of these changes are inevitable with age, you have a number of options available to you for preserving the health and vitality of your hair.

First, keep your hair trimmed to remove split, brittle ends and encourage volume. Some color treatments can give the effect of fullness and volumizing shampoos can coat thin hair to give it extra body. When you shampoo, use warm—not hot—water, and limit blow-drying as much as possible. Some deep conditioning treatments, used every few weeks, can help keep hair strong and less prone to breaking and splitting.

Your hair reflects your nutrition, too. Don't forget to include a wide variety of fresh fruit and vegetables in your diet, and take vitamin supplements to make sure that you're getting all of the recommended nutrients every day. Proper hydration is essential to healthy hair, so don't forget to drink the recommended thirty-two ounces or more of water every day.

Some prescription drugs are available to help manage menopausal hair problems:

- Minoxidil (marketed under the name Rogaine) works to stimulate hair follicles that may have grown dormant. Minoxidil can help restore lost hair by 10 percent or more, according to some estimates.

- Eflornithine may help stop unwanted hair growth. Eflornithine (marketed in its topical form as Vaniqa) can be applied as a cream directly to the area where unwanted hair growth occurs. The drug inhibits the production of an enzyme that contributes to hair growth; as a result, the drug slows the growth of unwanted hair.

 Alert

> Thinning, dry, brittle hair may be more than a natural sign of age. Some medications and certain systemic illnesses, such as a thyroid disorder, can also cause hair to lose its strength and vitality—even to the point of causing dramatic hair loss. Talk to your doctor or health care provider about noticeable changes to your hair's strength and appearance; don't assume it's simple aging.

Many of these hair and skin preparations and prescriptions take weeks, if not months, to show a result. Don't be discouraged and give up your treatment program if you don't see results overnight.

Making Time for Rest and Relaxation

Stress and fatigue are the enemies of your health, vitality, and natural beauty. Many of the most common symptoms of perimenopause and menopause are caused or complicated by excess stress and lack of rest. You may be accustomed to thinking of your body as a nonstop powerhouse that thrives on stress and performs best under pressure. Even if that belief held true when you were twenty, it doesn't hold true now. Your body and mind need adequate amounts of rest and enjoyment, especially during the years preceding menopause.

Participating in regular aerobic and strengthening exercise is critical for maintaining your body's ability to enjoy healthy, restful sleep. But part of your weekly fitness plan should also include some time—every day—for relaxation. Even thirty minutes of planned relaxation a day can make a big difference in your physical and mental health. Determine what relaxation technique works best for you—many activities can soothe your mind and rejuvenate feelings of well-being. Here are just a few suggestions:

- Mind/body practices, such as relaxation exercises, meditation, yoga, or Tai Chi
- Reading, listening to music, or playing an instrument
- Talking with friends, spending time with your partner, playing catch with your children, or walking your dog
- Soaking your feet, taking a leisurely bath, or giving yourself a facial
- Gardening, painting, or writing in a journal
- Reading religious texts or practicing your spiritual tradition

If your life is crowded, busy, and packed with a long to-do list or weighty responsibilities, you may need to force yourself to sit back, relax, and enjoy life for a few moments every day. But you won't look good, feel good, or perform well if you starve yourself of leisure. As you move through menopause, you have to consider rest and relaxation an essential component for a physically and emotionally healthy life.

 ## Fact

If you don't find positive ways to relax and reduce stress, you might find destructive ways to do so. Many people turn to food, alcohol, or drugs to help ease stress or avoid feelings of low self-esteem, anxiety, or boredom. When you feel that taking time for leisure and relaxation is an indulgence, remember what's at stake.

The menopausal period will bring both satisfying and challenging events. The better you take of yourself, the better able you are to meet them all head on. Although hormone issues and reproductive concerns may take center stage, you are a whole person who deserves proper attention.

Can Being Older Mean Being Happier?

CHAPTER 20

SOMETIMES WOMEN SEE MENOPAUSE as merely an entry into "old age." We live in a culture that makes fun of every decade after thirty by labeling it "over the hill." But what if menopause, like adolescence, is the doorway to a new and improved way of seeing the world? What if it is more of an opportunity than a disaster? What if, instead of the beginning of the end, it is the beginning of a beginning?

The Role of a Healthy Body and Mind

No one will argue that getting older brings some diminished physical capacities. There is a reason that athletes retire in their thirties, and as Lily Tomlin so aptly put it, "It's going to get worse before it gets worse." But today's aging population is more health conscious than any previous generation, and with advances in medicine and research every day, people learn how to age not only gracefully, but healthily. The quality of your life in middle age and beyond mostly depends on the condition of your body and general health. This book has given many suggestions and hints about how to make your body comfortable to live in, and the more you incorporate that thinking into your daily life, the better you will be able to enter this third age with confidence and ease.

The Role of Optimism

A healthy mind is more than just functioning brain tissue. Attitude and overall perspective can change your physiology, and make life more enjoyable. To paraphrase the Buddhists: Pain happens; suffering is optional. Research shows that your perceptions can determine your body's response to situations and to life. Optimistic people live longer and are less likely to become ill. The impact of optimism is profound, and can make all the difference in your quality of life as you age. And if you are thinking, "Well, it's just not me to be a Pollyanna," you may be right, but it *could* be you if you wanted it to be. Optimistic thinking patterns can be learned, and you can benefit from these shifts in perception, even if you have never been rosy by nature. The effect of changing your thoughts, as Eastern traditions have known for centuries, is that your body follows your thoughts. If you worry or perceive a situation as frightening, your body has a stress response to help you cope with the "danger." But if you train yourself to see situations as "puzzles" rather than "dangers," for example, your body has an entirely different response. Keeping your psyche out of the "danger" zone will make you much healthier as years go on.

 Alert

Pessimism can shorten your life! A study reported in the Journal of the American Medical Association describes a 2004 study showing that people who are optimistic by nature had a 23 percent lower risk of cardiovascular death, and 55 percent lower risk of death from all causes. To see whether you are optimistic or pessimistic, take one of the questionnaires on *www.authentichappiness.sas.upenn.edu.*

Your Vehicle Alters the Trip

When you take a long road trip, the vehicle you choose for your trip can make a big difference in how much you enjoy the ride. Similarly, when you make choices to keep your body healthy, your trip through middle age can be comfortable and enjoyable, or bumpy and painful. Your body is the only vehicle you have to carry your mind and spirit through your days, and the quality of the experience is directly related to how well you've maintained your "engine" and "chassis." This is not saying that you won't have repairs along the way, but if you can stay ahead of the problems and tend to them while they are small, you will get a lot more mileage out of your vehicle than you will if you wait until it is costly, or maybe impossible, to repair.

Fact

The MacArthur Study of Successful Aging followed a group of "successful agers" between the ages of seventy and seventy-nine for seven years. They found that the characteristics most highly associated with successful aging were exercise, social engagement, and a positive attitude. So if you want to postpone the effects of aging, stay active, affable, and upbeat.

Stress and Loss

Two inevitable forces that can age your beyond your years are stress and loss. As you deal with the stressors of life and grieve losses, it can take a toll on your health and well-being. Learning to find healthy coping strategies will not only extend your life but enhance it. There is no way to dodge either stress or loss, but there are plenty of ways to cope that lead to peace and resolution instead of anxiety and illness.

Coping with Stress

Stress is discussed in many places in this book, and for good reason. When you are under emotional or physical stress, your body produces hormones and chemicals to give you energy to deal with the stress. In the short run, this is a boost. But in the long run these chemicals are very hard on your body. We know that long-term stress can have the following effects:

- Stress can cause your blood pressure to rise.
- Stress can add to the likelihood of gaining "belly weight" which puts you at risk for heart disease.
- Stress can age your immune cells as much as ten years beyond other women your age who are not under stress, or who manage it better.
- Stress can damage your body's ability to regulate stress hormones, making them even more destructive to your system. Women are more prone to this "de-regulating" effect than men.

Essential

The title of the bestselling book by Richard Carlson probably describes the best approach to stress: *Don't Sweat the Small Stuff and It's All Small Stuff.* Keeping perspective when you are feeling overwhelmed is essential for staying well and sane. Remembering that, in the big picture, most irritations are "small stuff" is key to staying in balance. For hints about not sweating the small stuff, try *www .dontsweat.com.*

Your ability to manage stress is much better when you use stress reduction techniques. No one can escape the normal—or even the extraordinary—stressors that come in life, but you *can* learn to handle stress in ways that keep it from ruining your health, and aging you beyond your years.

Coping with Change and Loss

One characteristic of people who age successfully is the ability to cope with changes. And most difficult of all are changes associated with loss. As you experience more of life, you will necessarily experience more losses, including loss of physical abilities, parents, friends, pets, and other meaningful elements in your life. Other common losses and changes during this time are the loss of children to college or their own homes, the loss of income with retirement or divorce, the loss of partner through death or divorce, and the loss of a job with business restructuring or downsizing.

It is normal to grieve these losses, and it is also normal to develop coping strategies for managing the overwhelming feelings that are a part of grief response. Learning ways to cope that reduce anxiety and don't compromise your health are essential to healthy aging. If you turn to alcohol or chemicals to mask the sadness, they will harm your health and keep you from facing the emotional realities, thus prolonging your grief. People who rely on social supports and appropriate therapy are often the ones who bounce back and who have the fewest health problems resulting from these losses and changes.

Change and loss are part of life. Developing ways to deal with them prepares you to move flexibly into your middle age and beyond.

Alert

Grief is normal and can take a very long time to resolve. But "complicated," "unresolved," or "pathological" grief are all responses that require intervention. If you, or someone you know, has feelings of hurting themselves, chronic insomnia, overwhelming anxiety, ongoing emotional "numbness," or cannot function in everyday activities, make an appointment with a mental health professional right away for an evaluation.

Perspective Shifts after Fifty

What people sometimes call "midlife crisis" is actually a developmental shift in the way you see yourself and the world. It is common for people to become acutely aware of their own mortality sometime in midlife. Since this may be accompanied with other changes and losses, they may have the "time is running out" response and make dramatic changes in their lives, much to the astonishment and dismay of family and friends. If you see this as a normal shift in perspective, and avoid the panic responses of having an affair, changing jobs, or moving to a desert island, you can use this new perspective to design a life that is very satisfying.

Brain Development in Later Years

While some decline in your short-term (also called "working") memory is expected as you age, there are other changes that will actually make you a more flexible and adaptable thinker. The brain continues to grow cells, and the projections from these cells, called dendrites, grow and expand as the brain is challenged. That is why you need to exercise and challenge your brain as you get older—to grow more dendrite "branches." Along with the brain's tendency to transfer some activities to new parts of the brain when one area begins to fade, the net effect is one of overlap and communication that didn't happen when you were younger. In other words, your left brain is talking to your right brain in new and interesting patterns, helping you think in new ways. Your mind and heart are finally on the same page, or at least speaking the same language. This leads to all sorts of possibilities you have never considered. Whether it is an interpersonal problem at work or a special task like laying out the landscaping, you may be delighted to find that you are able to tackle processes that you used to find quite difficult.

Essential

With the increased communication between areas of the brain in midlife, many people begin to use "post formal" thought, which means that they understand the relative and non-absolute nature of knowledge. Once you begin to realize that many problems are not "black and white" but rather shades of gray, you will probably be more creative in problem solving.

Finding Meaning

As human development continues into midlife and beyond, you may find yourself assessing your values system. Over time, things that you have valued may seem somehow less important. If you were tied to possessions, status, or appearances, you may find yourself seeing a "bigger picture" and wanting to put your energy into something that will make a difference to the well-being of others. This is not a personality change; it is a developmental shift. Just as adolescents begin to think that toys are "silly," sometimes adults begin to wonder "what was I thinking?" about their previous choices or values. It is also common to notice an eagerness to find "meaning" in your life or work. It begins to make sense to you that you'd like to spend time at activities that have meaning beyond yourself or your family. This is a normal cognitive achievement, so give yourself permission to play with the possibilities. Older adults who find meaning in their work are more likely to stay engaged in life and thereby stay healthier as they age.

 Fact

> The Ontario Project on Successful Aging showed that the best predictor of happiness, perceived well-being, and absence of psychopathology and depression was "personal meaning." One of the researchers on the project, Dr. Paul T.P. Wong, states that "successful aging is 80 percent attitude, and 20 percent everything else." If that's the case, you have an 80 percent chance of determining whether you flourish as you get older.

Contributing to Your World

According to Dr. Gene Cohen, director of the Center on Aging, Health, and Humanities at George Washington University, age forty brings a developmental stage called "midlife evaluation." He describes this stage as a time of quest, where you consider where you've been and where you are going, and where you explore the opportunity to make course corrections to get where you want to be. Many people, men and women, find themselves thinking of their world in a broader sense. If you find yourself drawn to finding meaning by contributing to some larger entity, rest assured that you are developmentally right on track.

Defining Your "Contribution"

Women sometimes ask themselves at this stage, "Haven't I contributed enough? I've lived my whole life for other people." And in many cases this is true. Midlife is the time when your brain development and circumstances may offer you the first chance you've had to really examine where your contributions of time and energy go, and how you want to "spend" them. Instead of doing what you "have to" do, you can actually find things you "get to" do. Contributing can mean many things.

Maybe you have always played the piano, and now want to be part of a community theater group where your talent can be part of a larger effort. Or you have the time to join a quilting group that makes quilts for soldiers overseas. Maybe you like to write, and now you'd like to edit the newsletter for a local organization that you believe in. This may be the time when you volunteer with a church group going abroad to build safe water supplies in developing countries. Whatever your areas of interest, you may find yourself playing with ideas about how to pursue those interests and make a positive difference somewhere.

Fulfillment Opportunities

The next developmental phase is called the "liberation phase." This can be a very productive time of life, when people begin to ask, "If not now, when?" With brain development (dendrite growth) accelerating, people discover themselves solving problems in new ways, and—here's the great part—caring less and less what other people think! So it is an exciting convergence of mental ability and freedom from the conventional and cultural limits that have kept you from exploring. Since women are particularly sensitive to cultural expectations, they tend to experience this as unexpectedly freeing. Suddenly you are not concerned what the neighbors will think if you spend your vacation volunteering with the Red Cross or go off with a friend to an exotic location and rediscover who you really are.

Fulfillment is a personal thing, and what fulfills you might be unappealing to someone else. But during this phase of your life, you may find yourself excited about the endless possibilities for pushing the envelope. If you see this as a delightful and normal stage, you will be able to give yourself permission to define fulfillment in your own terms. You may find yourself explaining to friends and family (or yourself!) that you are not crazy. Indeed, you are just enjoying the liberation that comes with this new stage of life.

A New Kind of Intelligence

Given the changes in older brain development, experience, and social understanding, it is theorized that in midlife people develop a new, more integrated, system of interacting in the world. Researchers looking at brain plasticity—the ability to adapt and change in the face of challenges—are finding that as your brain compensates for some loss in cognitive tasks, you are developing whole new connections within your brain. These new ways of operating seem to integrate tasks that were previously managed separately, thus showing new perspectives. This process is probably the source of judgment and wisdom that were lacking in youth. You're not getting older, you're getting wiser!

Living for the Rest of Your Life

Menopause is a milepost on your path, but it is not the end of the line. The irregular periods or hot flashes may remind you that time is passing, and it is a perfect opportunity to consider where you've been in your life, and where you want to be in five or ten years. You can consider your physical fitness, your career, your family, and your social situation. Knowing the elements of healthy living, you can make decisions about where to go from here.

⌶ Essential

As you review your life situation, consider a technique used with depressed older adults: Radical Acceptance. Originally a Buddhist practice, radical acceptance has made its way into therapy circles via an innovative therapy used with suicidal patients. It means accepting things as they are—just as they are—without judging or changing them. It frees up energy for problem solving that you may be using for regret, disappointment, or resentment.

Reviewing the Story So Far

One of the developmental tasks of midlife is to make sense of your life to this point. It is the ideal moment to decide what you've done well, and what you'd like to improve. Later you will go through a stage where you may feel a need to do a "life review." But in midlife, beginning around forty, you may want to take stock and decide if you are on the road you want to be. It is stimulating and emotionally healthy to play with possibilities and try on new or different roles for yourself.

Making a Plan

If you determine that there is some goal you've never been able to achieve, and you'd like to begin walking toward it, sit down and make a plan. Are there courses you could take that would prepare you? Travel plans you could explore? Books that would inform you about how to reach that target? Even if your life is crammed with responsibilities, you might find it enjoyable and satisfying to plan toward a lifelong (maybe secret) ambition.

Whether it is a trip to Eastern Europe or a career in real estate, if you have an undying desire for a new or different direction, you could begin planning for it now. Treat it as a research project, or see it as your little escape. Sit down in a quiet moment and write down the three steps that would get you closer to your goal. Even planning can lift your spirits and build excitement for something new. Is there a club you could join where people could help you think about your dream?

 Fact

It's never too late to set goals. Research has shown that performance is enhanced by setting goals. In other words, once you set goals you are much more likely to accomplish something than if you just think about it, and don't set goals. This is true for both younger and older adults. So grab a pen and jot down what you're aiming at—you'll probably make it!

What Goals Make Sense for You?

If you do have a lifelong or new ambition, decide whether this is a fantasy dream or a real possibility. Then outline the goals that are achievable. Talk to friends about your wish. Discuss it with your spouse or partner. They may have ideas about how to incorporate it into your life. You may find there are ways to pursue a new direction that are very manageable in your current lifestyle.

And if you are considering a major change, let your family in on it and ask for their help in making it come true. Can you go to night school to become an accountant? Have you always wanted to go to nursing school? What would it take to learn SCUBA diving? Talk these possibilities over with close friends and family and get their feedback on what is reasonable. This is your chance to realize a dream while you are young, healthy, and eager to learn.

Be Creative!

Even if you don't have an undying desire to change your career or travel the world, you may find yourself thinking of ways to express your creativity. Your brain is continuing to develop, and challenging it with creative pursuits is a great way to stay engaged in your life. If you have a hobby you'd like to expand, or a skill you'd like to learn, that is completely in line with your developmental stage.

"I'm Not the Creative Type"

You may not think of yourself as creative, but there are many ways to express your creativity and lots of support to do so. Dr. Howard Gardner, a noted Harvard developmental psychologist, distinguishes between Creativity with a capital "C" and creativity with a small "c." Big "C" Creativity is the type of breakthrough, well-known creativity of extraordinary people. Albert Einstein, Mozart, Mother Theresa, and Gandhi, for example, used unconventional and creative ways of thinking to transform the world. But small "c" creativity is available to everyone. It is about taking the risk of breaking routine or convention to try something original. It could be planting a garden where you've always wanted one; writing a letter to someone you've never communicated with; starting a lunchtime book group or a walking club at work. Whatever you feel drawn to, and have not explored, that is an entrée into creativity for you. Anyone who challenges his or her mind to try something new or unusual is walking down a creative road.

Beyond the Craft Store

Spend some time thinking about where your strengths and interests lie. Are you involved in those things through your work? Or have you used hobbies to explore those areas? If not, why not take some steps toward engaging in activities that stimulate and intrigue you. Here are some ideas for starters, but of course you will have your own:

- Take up folk dancing.
- Join a local theater group—even as a volunteer if you want to get your feet wet.
- Learn a new computer skill.
- Try digital photography.
- Do an internship with a professional in your area of interest.
- Volunteer as a mentor.

It hardly matters what your area of interest is, there are ways to include it in your life. Whether your passion is children or Italian opera, you can create ways to explore it and share your skill and interest with others. Recipe clubs, cross country skiing, or knitting klatches all offer the chance to create something new in your world, and you will be healthier and happier for it.

 Fact

In a famous quote by Confucius, dating from about 500 B.C., he noted, "At fifteen I set my heart upon learning. At thirty I established myself in accordance with ritual. At forty I no longer had perplexities. At fifty I knew the mandate of heaven. At sixty I was at ease with whatever I heard. At seventy I could follow my heart's desire without transgressing the boundaries of right."

The Real Creation—You

Menopause is a life-changing event. It offers opportunity along with the physical changes, and brings the prospect of going from "reproductive" to "productive." It is a chance to become more of who you are, and more of who you are meant to be. Although you will undoubtedly be faced with challenges—physical, emotional, and spiritual—you decide every day and every minute how to respond to those challenges. Those decisions will create the most important thing you have to offer the world: yourself. Being older can mean being happier. And it can mean finally being you.

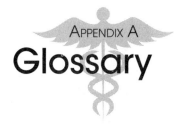

APPENDIX A

Glossary

A

Amenorrhea
A cessation or absence of menstrual periods.

Androgens
Male hormones normally produced in small quantities by the female ovaries and adrenal glands, with the greatest quantities occurring at the midpoint of a woman's menstrual cycle. Androgens are thought to promote a healthy sex drive and are sometimes prescribed as part of a full regimen of hormone replacement therapy.

Andropause
See Male Menopause.

Angina
A squeezing, heaviness, or tightness in your chest that happens when your heart muscle is deprived of oxygen.

Antioxidants
Certain vitamins, including vitamins A, C, E, and beta carotene, found in some brightly colored fruits and vegetables, considered to be important tools in warding off heart disease and

some cancers and may even reduce age-related macular degeneration or AMD (age-related vision loss).

Atherosclerosis
A blood vessel condition that develops when the buildup of plaque on arterial walls narrows the arterial passage and thus limits the amount of blood that can flow through the arteries to nourish the heart, brain, kidneys, and other organs.

B

Biofeedback
A technique in which individuals are trained to control any bodily function by recognizing feedback from that body function enough to learn to control it. For example, people can monitor their breathing, heart rate, and blood pressure (with the use of various instruments), then change the rate of those functions through relaxation techniques or visual imagery.

Bioflavonoids
Naturally occurring plant substances found in many brightly colored fruits and vegetables, such as cherries, oranges, other citrus, grapes, leafy

291

vegetables, wine, and some types of red clover. Bioflavonoids are being studied for the treatment of a number of conditions, including the control of bleeding, hemorrhoids, and varicose veins.

BMI (body mass index)

A measurement of a person's percentage of fat, determined by dividing a person's weight by his or her height.

C

Calcitonin

A hormone produced by the parathyroid gland to help regulate calcium levels in the bloodstream, and in so doing, protect bone density. Calcitonin is available in prescription form for the treatment of postmenopausal osteoporosis.

Cardiovascular Disease

A term used to describe a variety of heart diseases, illnesses, and events affecting the heart and circulatory system, including high blood pressure and coronary artery disease.

Chemotherapy

The use of potent medications to treat cancer, usually by affecting cells that are rapidly growing, such as the cancer cells themselves.

Coronary Artery Disease

A common form of heart disease that results when the heart receives inadequate amounts of oxygen-rich blood through its arteries. This disease usually occurs when arteries become lined with heavy deposits of plaque—a substance made up of fat and calcium in a condition known as atherosclerosis.

D

Dendrites

The fine appendages at the ends of brain cells that transmit brain signals.

Dehydroepiandrosterone (DHEA)

An important hormone in the female body that decreases as a woman ages and declines dramatically after menopause. DHEA is thought to combat memory and bone loss, and it may help to maintain breast and cardiovascular health.

DHEA

See Dehydroepiandrosterone (DHEA).

E

Endometrial Cancer

Cancer of the endometrium.

Endometrial Hyperplasia

An overgrowth of the lining of the uterus that can be precancerous but is not always. It is typically diagnosed through a biopsy or sampling of the uterine lining, a procedure most doctors perform in their office.

Endometrium

The lining of the uterus.

Endorphins

Naturally occurring substances released by the brain that resemble opiates and are considered to be the brain chemicals that make you feel happy and content.

Estradiol
The main form of estrogen produced by the ovaries, and the body's most efficient and potent estrogen.

Estrogen
A class of female sex hormones produced by the ovaries, pituitary gland, and (in small quantities) by body fat. During puberty, estrogen stimulates the development of adult sex organs and the adult female breasts, hips, and buttocks. Estrogen helps to retain calcium in bones, regulates the balance of HDL and LDL cholesterol in the bloodstream and aids the maintenance of blood sugar level, memory functions, and emotional balance.

F

Fibroids
Benign growths of muscle cells that develop within or on the uterine wall.

Follicle-Stimulating Hormone (FSH)
Produced by the pituitary gland, promotes follicle development within the ovary, thus allowing certain eggs to mature and the follicle cells surrounding each egg to produce estrogen in preparation for fertilization.

FSH
See Follicle-Stimulating Hormone (FSH).

H

HDL Cholesterol
The high-density lipoprotein fraction of cholesterol ("good" cholesterol) that helps prevent heart disease by breaking up and carrying the low-density lipoprotein (LDL cholesterol) out of the bloodstream and into the liver for metabolism and evacuation in the feces.

Heart Palpitations
The uncomfortable sensation that the heart is beating rapidly, out of sequence, too strenuously, or in some other abnormal fashion.

Hippocampus
The part of the brain responsible for creating, storing, and retrieving memory.

Hormone Replacement Therapy (HRT)
Therapy consisting of estrogen or a combination of estrogen and progestin designed to replace the loss of these hormones in menopause and thus combat the effects of this deficiency, including bone loss, vaginal atrophy, hot flashes, and other conditions. See also Menopause Hormone Therapy (MHT).

Hot Flashes (Flushes)
Hot flashes or flushes can be mild or severe, but in general, they involve a fast-spreading sensation of warmth through the face, neck, and shoulders. Hot flashes are the result of fluctuating hormone levels, but their

triggers, intensity, and frequency vary from woman to woman. Hot flashes that occur during sleep are often known as night sweats.

HRT
See Hormone Replacement Therapy (HRT).

Hypertension
High blood pressure that occurs when arteries become too inflexible to allow an ample supply of blood to circulate, especially under periods of exertion or stress, thus causing excess pressure against arterial walls. Severe or ongoing high blood pressure can lead to damage of the body organs, including stroke and other life-threatening conditions.

Hysterectomy
The surgical removal of the uterus, which may or may not also be accompanied by the removal of the cervix and/or ovaries. If ovaries remain, the hysterectomy doesn't necessarily cause menopause, though menstrual bleeding ceases.

I

Induced Menopause
A cessation of menstrual cycles that occurs when a woman has her ovaries surgically removed in a procedure called oophorectomy, or when a woman's ovaries cease to function prematurely as a result of medication, radiation, or disease. With treatment and intervention, some non-surgical types of induced menopause may be temporary. See also Temporary Menopause.

Insomnia
An inability to fall and/or remain asleep that occurs three or more nights a week.

Isoflavones
A type of plant estrogen found in soybeans, red clover, and (in much lower quantities) green tea, peas, pinto beans, lentils, and other legumes, that may have benefits in treating some symptoms of menopause.

K

Kegel Exercise
An exercise designed to strengthen the muscles of the pelvic floor to improve vaginal muscle tone, enhance sexual response, and limit involuntary urine release due to stress urinary incontinence.

L

LDL Cholesterol
Low-density lipoprotein cholesterol ("bad" cholesterol) is transported through the arteries by a complex of lipids and proteins. In high concentrations, this cholesterol is associated with an increased risk of atherosclerosis and coronary heart disease.

LH
See Luteinizing Hormone (LH).

Luteinizing Hormone (LH)
A hormone produced by the pituitary gland, LH has multiple functions, one of which is prompting ovulation.

M

Major Depression
An emotional disorder characterized by extreme or prolonged feelings of sadness, despair, guilt, or hopelessness so debilitating that they affect one's normal quality of life and/or work performance.

Male Menopause
Known as andropause in the medical community, male menopause is associated with an age-related decrease in male hormone levels in men; symptoms can include lethargy, depression, mood swings, insomnia, hot flashes, irritability, and decreased sexual desire and function.

Mammogram
A low-dose X-ray of the breast used to screen for or examine lumps that may signify breast cancer.

Menarche
The first menstrual period.

Menopause
The permanent end of menstruation and fertility. See also Natural Menopause, Induced Menopause, and Temporary Menopause.

Menopause Hormone Therapy (MHT)
Using a combination of hormones to treat the symptoms of decreasing estrogen and progesterone. The hormones may include estrogen, progestin, and variations of either, alone or in combination. See also Hormone Replacement Therapy (HRT).

Migraine Headaches
Intensely painful headaches thought to be associated with spasms that constrict blood vessels in the brain. Women who suffer migraines describe them as pounding headaches that can produce nausea, vomiting, and a painful sensitivity to light, noise, and odors.

N

Natural Menopause
The cessation of all periods resulting from the halt of ovarian hormone production that is spontaneous and not the result of other physical or pathological conditions or treatments; natural menopause is diagnosed when a women has had twelve months of amenorrhea.

Night Sweats
See Hot Flashes.

Nutraceuticals
Although no legally determined or internationally accepted definition exists for this term, in the marketplace the term is used to describe foods or dietary supplements that claim to deliver some sort of medication or compound designed to offer a specific medical benefit.

O

Obesity
A condition of being more than 30 percent over your ideal weight, or

having a body mass index (BMI) of 25 or higher.

Omega-3 Fatty Acids

Essential fatty acids, found in cold-water fatty fish, nuts, flaxseed, tofu, and in soybean and canola oils, that help nourish the hair and nails and offer a number of benefits for cardiovascular health.

Oophorectomy

The surgical removal of one or both ovaries.

Osteoporosis

The reduction in bone density 2.5 standard deviations below the average bone density of a thirty-year-old woman. This loss of bone mass results in porous, fragile bone that is prone to fracture. An age-related disease in menopause, osteoporosis can manifest itself sooner in women who have risk factors.

Ovulation

The release of a mature egg from a properly developed ovarian follicle.

P

Pap Smear

A cell sample taken (as a swab) during an internal vaginal exam to test for precancerous cell changes and cervical cancer.

Perimenopause

The period of transition to natural menopause during which the body undergoes endocrinologic and biologic changes resulting from declin-ing ovarian hormone production; symptoms can include irregular menstrual periods, hot flashes, vaginal dryness, insomnia, and mood swings. Perimenopause is highly variable and can last many years (four years is average), and ends after twelve months of amenorrhea.

Phytohormones

Natural substances found in some herbs and other plants that may help to regulate plant growth. Some types, referred to as phytoestrogens, can bind to the human body's estrogen receptors and may act like an estrogen or an anti-estrogen on the body, depending upon their particular type and dosage.

PMDD

See Premenstrual Dysphoric Disorder (PMDD).

PMS

See Premenstrual Syndrome (PMS).

Polyp, Uterine

Small, tag-shaped growths of uterine tissue, attached to the lining of the uterus. Polyps can cause irregular bleeding; doctors remove them to confirm there is no precancerous change.

Premenstrual Dysphoric Disorder (PMDD)

A debilitating premenstrual syndrome that can include symptoms such as severe depression, anxiety, sleep disturbances, and fatigue in addition to a wide range of physical disturbances. Though premenstrual syndrome (PMS) and PMDD differ in severity, diagnosis, and treatment, both seem to be linked to the way the body processes and responds to reproductive hormones and possibly to serotonin.

Premenstrual Syndrome (PMS)
A condition occurring ten to fourteen days before the onset of menstrual bleeding and involving physical and emotional symptoms that include bloating, water retention, pelvic pressure or cramping, headaches or migraines, irritability, mood swings, difficulty concentrating, and food cravings.

Progesterone
A female sex hormone, produced in largest amounts during and after ovulation, that prepares the uterus for the implantation of a fertilized egg.

Progestin
A chemical name for various types of synthetic progesterone. Progestin is used in HRT to balance the effects of estrogen on the endometrium and prevent endometrial hyperplasia and cancer.

S

Selective Estrogen Receptor Modulators (SERMs)
A class of drugs that act like estrogens on some body tissues and anti-estrogens in other body tissues. They are being studied for possible roles in both prevention of bone loss

(an estrogen-like action in the bone) and reduction of breast cancer risk (an anti-estrogen type action in the breast). Raloxifene is one example of a SERM.

SERM
See Selective Estrogen Receptor Modulators (SERMs).

Statins
Cholesterol-lowering drugs.

Stress Urinary Incontinence
The unpredictable and involuntary loss of urine caused by weakened sphincter muscles (the muscles that surround the urethra) and often triggered by an event such as a sneeze or cough.

T

Temporary Menopause
An interruption of the ovarian function that prevents the production of hormones that accompany the maturation and release of oocytes (eggs). Temporary menopause can follow chemical or radiation therapies or disease. When the contributing condition stops, ovulation and menstruation begin again. See also Induced Menopause.

Triglycerides
A type of fat found in the blood; other types of this fat include butter, margarine, and vegetable oil. Triglyceride levels are checked in total fasting lipid profiles (blood tests, sometimes called coronary panels,

that check levels of HDL cholesterol, LDL cholesterol, and triglycerides).

U

Urethra
The tubular structure connecting the bladder to the outside of the body allowing the bladder to empty.

Urge Incontinence
The loss of urine associated with the urge to void. The urge may be triggered by water, key in the lock (anticipating entry to the bathroom), or by nothing.

Urinary Incontinence
See Stress Urinary Incontinence.

Urinary Tract Infections (UTI)
Upper or lower tract infection of the bladder or kidney, or both. Bacterial infections in the bladder result from ascending bacteria from the perineum, especially when defenses are lowered. Another common cause of bacterial infections is the urethral atrophy that often occurs after menopause.

UTI
See Urinary Tract Infections (UTI).

V

Vaginal Atrophy
A condition characterized by the thinning and flattening of the vaginal wall. The decreased total surface area of the vagina leads to decreased transudate secretions, and this leads to vaginal dryness. Over time, the vaginal wall becomes less flexible

and can actually shrink and these changes can lead to the risk of tears or cracking.

Vaginitis
An inflammation of the vagina. It may be due to infection from bacteria, yeast, or other pathogens, resulting in discomfort, itching, and/or abnormal discharge.

Vasomotor Symptoms
Hot flashes or night sweats that result from hormonal fluctuations in menopause and perimenopause.

Keeping a Menopause Journal

A menopause journal can be an important tool for both you and your doctor. By chronicling your experiences, you create a clear vision of the physical and emotional changes you've experienced to help you understand where you've been—and perhaps, where you're going—as you move into the final third of your life.

Your Journal as a Medical Record

You keep a menopause journal to record the physical and emotional symptoms you experience each day as you move toward and through menopause. Part of your journal will be a medical record, where you list physical observations, such as migraine headaches, irregular periods, sleepless nights, changes in your weight, and so on. This same calendar should include your menstrual periods, so that if an association exists, you or your doctor will be able to notice. You aren't just keeping a record of your symptoms, but of their severity, frequency, and recurrence—so you can spot any patterns that occur.

Your doctors can gauge your response to medications and other treatment options you're exploring. If certain symptoms occur in tandem or in a specific sequence each month, especially in conjunction with your periods, or with a lack of menstrual bleeding, that information may explain the specific triggering mechanism that prompts them.

Your Journal as a Personal Record

You also can use your journal to record your emotional symptoms and responses to the process of passing through perimenopause and menopause. The very act of writing down your thoughts and feelings is a powerful tool for understanding them. Your journal gives you a much closer look at who you are, who you're becoming, what you most fear, and what your hopes for the future entail. And, the accurate record of the progress and patterns of your symptoms over the months in your journal actually can help you manage your reactions to some menopausal symptoms and expand your understanding of the process you're experiencing.

For example, your journal may record anxiety attacks, and over time, you realize that those that wake you up at 3 A.M. and cost you hours of sleepless worry occur most often between the tenth through fourteenth days of your cycle. This understanding may enable you to say to yourself, "This panic I'm feeling is a chemical response to hormonal fluctuations, not a true reaction to impending disaster." With that, you may be able to do your deep breathing exercises, calm your mind, and return to sleep more quickly.

If you suffer from stress, simply writing in your journal may give you a means for lessening the effects of this health-eroding condition. By writing about your stress—events that triggered the stress, your reactions, and your thoughts about resolving the stress-inducing issues in your life—you give yourself a moment to stop the cycle of nervous tension, worry, anger, and fear that add fuel and momentum to your stress.

Many women have noted that perimenopause and menopause trigger feelings of introspection they haven't experienced before. If you find yourself thinking about your past, recollecting family vacations, relatives you haven't seen for years, or your old boyfriends, write it down! These thoughts and ideas are important to you right now, or they wouldn't be occupying your mind. Making a record of them helps you take a broader look at exactly what about these past events may be saying to you now. Just remember to keep separate medical and personal journals, or transfer information from one journal into the symptom diary or calendar that you plan to take with you to your doctor's appointments.

Important Medical Information to Note

What kind of medical information and records do you want to maintain in your journal? This book has discussed the types of symptoms your doctor may want you to record in a monthly symptom diary. Most such records include a list, by the day of your menstrual cycle, of symptoms experienced, and the severity of those symptoms (usually noted as mild, moderate, or severe). Some typical symptoms included in symptom diaries or calendars are mood swings, irritability, insomnia, hot flashes, night sweats, weight change, headache, increased appetite, fatigue, depression, and forgetfulness. When you're preparing to begin your menopause journal, talk to your doctor to find out what symptoms he or she would most like for you to track over the next few months.

Though your menopause journal is much more than just this list of physical and emotional symptoms, those records are an important source of information for both you and your doctor, so choose them carefully. Here are some ideas:

- **Keep a diet journal.** List the foods you eat, serving sizes, and calorie counts if you're concerned about tracking the source of weight gain you may be experiencing or improving your nutrition. Many women have no idea how much they eat during the day, or how well their diet conforms to the recommendations set forward by most health experts. (See Chapter 13 for more information on those guidelines.)

- **Keep an exercise journal.** When you note the type of exercise you do each day, the length of time you exercise, number of repetitions, and related information, you'll be able to track your progress and note any associations between your exercise, your symptoms, weight changes, and overall feelings of well-being.

- **Track all cyclical symptoms.** Many women experience cyclical symptoms as they move through perimenopause. For example, hot flashes, migraine headaches, or insomnia may occur at specific points in the menstrual cycles. Your symptom calendar will help you track these recurring symptoms. Don't just be on high alert for negative days; track those positive feelings as well. Your "up" days may occur on a regular basis, and could provide you and your doctor with important information about hormone cycles, diet, or other factors that contribute to them.

- **Note changes in medication or supplements.** You don't need to begin each day's journal entry with a list of all of the vitamins and routine medications you've taken on that day; one entry in your journal should include that list, for the record. But note any changes from your daily routine; add and remove medications as your prescriptions change or end, and note changes in the types or amounts of vitamin and mineral supplements you're taking. If you switch from brand-name prescriptions to generic, record that, too.

Appendix C

References and Resources

Print and Online Articles, Journals, and Magazines

Jacobs Institute of Women's Health Expert Panel on Menopause Counseling "Guidelines for Counseling Women on the Management of Menopause." Jacobs Institute of Women's Health, online, *www.jiwh.org*.

National Women's Health Information Center. "Menopause and Menopause Treatments, Frequently Asked Questions." U.S. Department of Health and Human Services, Office on Women's Health, March, 2006.

National Institutes of Health. "NIH State-of-the-Science Conference Statement on Management of Menopause-Related Symptoms." National Institutes of Health. March, 2005.

deBruin, J.P., et al. "The Role of Genetic Factors in Age at Natural Menopause." *Human Reproduction*. European Society of Human Reproduction and Embryology. September, 2001.

North American Menopause Society. "Menopause Guidebook: Helping Women Make Informed Healthcare Decisions Around Menopause and Beyond." North American Menopause Society. October, 2006. *www. menopause.org/edumaterials/ guidebook/mgtoc.htm*.

Hitti, Miranda. "Antiseizure Drug May Ease Hot Flashes." WebMD Health News, July, 2006. *www.medscape.com*.

Sicat, Brigitte L. and Deborah K. Brokaw. "Nonhormonal Alternatives for the Treatment of Hot Flashes." *Pharmacotherapy*, 2004. Pharmacotherapy Publications.

Carroll, Dana G. "Nonhormonal Therapies for Hot Flashes in Menopause." *American Family Physician*, February, 2006.

Busko, Marlene. "Physical Fitness Contributes to Successful Mental Aging." Medscape Medical News, October, 2006. *www.medscape.com.*

Mieszkowski, Katharine. "Which Cancer Kills the Most American Women?" Salon.com, Salon Media Group Inc. November, 2006. *www.salon.com.*

National Cancer Institute. "A Snapshot of Breast Cancer." September, 2006. *http://planning. cancer.gov/disease/snapshots.*

National Health, Lung and Blood Institute. "WISE Study of Women and Heart Disease Yields Important Findings on Frequently Undiagnosed Syndrome." *NIH News.* National Institutes of Health, January, 2006.

Gavin, Kara. "Post-Stroke Tests Not Used Often Enough, Especially in Women, U-M Study Finds." University of Michigan Health System, September, 2005. *www.med .umich.edu/opm/newspage/ 2005/womenstroke.htm.*

American Academy of Family Physicians. "Heart Disease and Heart Attacks: What Women Need to Know." Online Handout. October, 2005. *http:// familydoctor.org/287.xml.*

American Heart Association. "ACC/AHA Guidelines for the Management of Patients with Valvular Heart Disease – General Principles. A Report of the American College of Cardiology/ American Heart Association Task Force on Practice Guidelines." American Heart Association, 1998. *www.americanheart.org.*

National Center for Complementary and Alternative Medicine. "Could CAM Therapies Help Menopausal Symptoms?" Backgrounder. National Institutes of Health, November, 2005. Public Domain.

National Institutes of Health. "Phytoestrogens and Bone Health." NIH Osteoporosis and Related Bone Diseases—National Resource Center, August, 2005.

Lee, Dennis. "Migraine Headache." MedicineNet.com, July, 2002. *www.medicinenet.com/ migraine_headache/article.htm.*

Krahn, Lois. "Which Came First: Insomnia, Depression, or Menopause?" Practical Strategies in Women's Health, Fall, 2006.

Brown, Marie-Annett, et al. "The Effects of a Multi-Modal Intervention Trial of Light, Exercise and

Vitamins on Women's Mood."
Woman & Health, 34(3), 2001.

Jacoby, Susan. "Sex in America."
AARP The Magazine. August,
2005. *www.aarpmagazine.org/*
*lifestyle/relationships/sex_in_*
america.html.

Mayo Clinic Staff. "Female
Sexual Dysfunction." Mayo-
Clinic.com. April, 2006 *www*
.mayoclinic.com/health/female
-sexual-dysfunction/DS00701.

Books on Menopause, Women's Health, and Aging

American Medical Association.
The American Medical Associa-
tion Complete Guide to Women's
Health. (New York, N.Y: Random House, Inc., 1996).

Boston Women's Health
Collective. *Our Bodies, Our-*
selves: Menopause. 1st Ed.
(New York, NY: Touchstone/
Simon & Schuster, 2006).

Cohen, Gene D. *The Creative*
Age: Awakening Human Poten-
tial in the Second Half of Life.
(New York, NY: Harper/Collins
Publishers, 2000).

DeAngelis, Lissa and Molly Siple.
Recipes for Change: Gourmet

Wholefood Cooking for Health
and Vitality at Menopause.
(New York, NY: Dutton Books,
1996).

Greer, Germaine. *The Change:*
Women, Aging, and the
Menopause. (New York, NY:
Alfred A. Knopf, 1992).

Nelson, Miriam and Sarah
Wernick. *Strong Women*
Stay Young.(New York, NY:
Bantam Books, 2005).

Northrup, Christiane. *The*
Wisdom of Menopause: Creat-
ing Physical and Emotional
Health and Healing During the
Change. (New York, NY: Ban-
tam Doubleday Dell, 2001).

Seligman, Martin E. *Learned*
Optimism: How to Change
Your Mind and Your Life. (New
York, NY: Vintage Books/
Random House, 2006).

Sheehy, Gail. *The Silent Passage:*
Menopause, rev. ed. (New York,
NY: Random House, 1998).

Web Resources

Exercise

Yoga
www.yoga.com

Tai Chi

✐www.arthritis.org/
resources/arthritistoday/2000_
archives/2000_07_08_taichi.asp
✐www.aarp.org/health/fitness/
work_out/Articles/a2003-08-29-
martialarts.html

Walkingprograms

✐http://walking.about.com/
od/howtowalk
✐www.aarp.org/health/fitness
/walking
✐www.cdc.gov/nccdphp/dnpa/
physical/health_professionals/
active_environments/aces.htm

Pilates

✐www.pilatesinsight.com

Incontinence

✐http://kidney.niddk.nih
.gov/kudiseases/pubs/pdf/
menopause_ez.pdf

Hot Flashes

✐http://nccam.nih.gov/health

Organizations

The American Association of Retired Persons (AARP)

601 E Street NW
Washington, D.C. 20049
✐www.aarp.org

The American Cancer Society (ACS)

800-ACS-2345
✐www.cancer.org

American College of Obstetricians and Gynecologists (ACOG)

409 12th Street SW
Washington, DC 20024-2188
202-638-5577
✐wwww.acog.org

AmericanDiabetes Association (ADA)

1701 N. Beauregard Street
Alexandria, VA 22311
800-342-2383
✐www.diabetes.org

TheAmerican Heart Association (AHA)

7272 Greenville Avenue
Dallas, TX 75231
800-AHA-USA1
✐www.americanheart.org

The American Lung Association (ALA)

1740 Broadway
New York, NY 10019
800-LUNG-USA
✐www.lungusa.org

**The American Menopause
Foundation (AMF)**
350 Fifth Avenue, Suite 2822
New York, NY 10119
212-714-2398
www.americanmenopause.org

**The American Psychiatric
Association (APA)**
1400 K Street NW
Washington, DC 20005
888-357-7924
www.psych.org

**American Society for Repro-
ductive Medicine (ASRM)**
1209 Montgomery Highway
Birmingham, AL 35216-2809
205-978-5000
www.asrm.org

**The Association of Repro-
ductive Health Profes-
sionals (ARHP)**
2401 Pennsylvania Avenue NW
Suite 350
Washington, DC 20037
800-804-7374
www.arhp.org

**Food and Nutrition
Information Center**
Agricultural Research
Service, USDA
National Agricultural
Library, Room 105
10301 Baltimore Avenue
Beltsville, MD 20705-2351

301-504-5719
www.nal.usda.gov/fnic

**National Association for
Continence (NAFC)**
P.O. Box 1019
Charleston, SC 29402-1019
800-BLADDER
www.nafc.org

**International Council on
Active Aging (ICAA)**
3307 Trutch Street
Vancouver, BC, V6L-2T3
866-335-9777
604-734-4466
www.icaa.cc/Aboutus.htm

**The National Cancer
Institute (NCI)**
Bldg. 31, Room 10A31
31 Center Drive, MSC 2580
Bethesda, MD 20892-2580
800-4-CANCER
www.nci.nih.gov

**The National Center for
Complementary and Alter-
native Medicine (NCCAM)**
NCCAM Clearinghouse
P.O. Box 7923
Gaithersburg, MD 20898
888-644-6226
301-519-3153
E-mail: info@nccam.nig.gov
http://nccam.nih.gov

National Institute on Aging (NIA)

Building 31, Room 5C27
31 Center Drive, MSC 2292
Bethesda, MD 20892
✐*www.nia.nih.gov*

National Institute of Diabetes and Digestive and Kidney Diseases (NIDDK)

NIDDK, NIH,
Building 31, Room 9A04
31 Center Drive, MSC 2560
Bethesda, MD 20892-2560
✐*www.niddk.nih.gov*

National Osteoporosis Foundation (NOF)

1232 22nd Street NW
Washington, DC 20037-1292
202-223-2226
✐*www.nof.org*

The National Sleep Foundation (NSF)

1522 K Street NW, Suite 500
Washington, DC 20005
202-347-3471
✐*www.sleepfoundation.org*

National Women's Health Information Center

U.S. Department of Health
and Human Services
The North American Menopause
Society (NAMS)
P.O. Box 94572
Cleveland, OH 44101
440-442-7550
✐*www.menopause.org*

Office on Women's Health

U.S. Department of Health
and Human Services
200 Independence Avenue, SW
Room 712E
Washington, D.C. 20201
202-690-7650
800-994-9662
TDD 888-220-5446
✐*http://womenshealth.gov*

Your After-Forty Health Maintenance Plan

Okay, you've reviewed some of the health issues that you need to keep in mind after age forty and know how to put together your family and personal health histories. All of this information lays the foundation for building a strong, effective health plan that will help you and your health care provider keep tabs on your health in the years ahead. Some commonsense lifestyle guidelines and regular medical examinations are your ticket to a comfortable, healthy middle age.

To get started, find a small calendar with room for notes, and jot down one or two goals for each month. Choose from any of the following categories. Don't overwhelm yourself with good intentions—make no more than two goals per month, and dedicate yourself to giving them a real try for the full month. Four weeks of a new activity is often enough to internalize it so that it becomes part of your routine.

Diet

With the information in Chapter 16 of this book, or any reasonable, well-rounded diet plan, you can make a big difference in your overall well-being. Find one small diet goal each month, and incorporate it into your routine. After a year, you will have several new eating habits that support your health. Consider one of these for each month:

- Replace one high fat item with its low-fat equivalent (cheese, milk, meat—whichever is easiest to start with).
- Add one serving per day of colorful vegetables.
- Add two glasses of water to your daily intake.
- Hide the saltshaker.
- Wean yourself off of caffeine drinks.
- Add one serving of fish per week to your dinner menus.

- Eat breakfast every day.
- Drop sugar from your diet for a month and see how you feel.
- Keep a food diary—sometimes awareness of what you are eating is revealing about what you need to change.

If you change your diet in even five or six small ways by the end of a year, you are making progress toward a healthier lifestyle.

Exercise

If you are making small changes, you are more likely to keep them up. On your "Health Maintenance Calendar," choose exercise goals that are very small and reasonable. It's best to take it very slowly, so you don't get discouraged, so add an exercise goal about every other month or so. Here are some ideas to get you started:

- Choose one activity that you really love. Walking, swimming, biking, dancing—whatever is fun for you and accessible. Find a way to do it for twenty minutes at least three times a week for a month. Mark it on the calendar when you do the activity, and notice how you feel at the end of the month.
- Take the stairs at work.
- Try an activity that you've always wanted to, or know you enjoy, with a buddy. Ask a work friend to walk on your lunch hour, take salsa dancing with a friend, go kayaking, bike around a lake. Just give your body something new to do, and mark it on your calendar.
- Walk around the block every day at lunchtime.
- Incorporate some stretching routine for a month. Take a Tai Chi class or do yoga for fifteen minutes in the morning, up to three times a day.

If you start using your body more than you have in the past, it will start to respond and "ask" you to move more. The combination of small diet changes and small activity changes can make you feel better even if your weight remains constant.

Emotional Well-being

Your emotional well-being is critical for maintaining your health. You can learn skills and take some steps toward a more emotionally healthy life whether you are already pretty balanced and happy or seek to become more so. By incorporating simple things into a monthly health maintenance plan, you can change your outlook and emotional state. Here are some possibilities:

- Keep a gratitude journal. It's easy to lose sight of the many positives in your life, and jotting them down once a day keeps things in perspective.
- Do one spontaneous kind act each day. A secret gift left on the desk of a coworker; take an aging neighbor out for lunch; keep dollars in your pocket for homeless people. Once you are looking for a daily "kindness quota," opportunities will abound.
- Read a book about learned optimism or positive psychology and try it out. Changing the way you think can change your physiology—for the better!
- Get counseling. If you are persistently feeling negative or as though you are not emotionally okay, this will take a toll on your health. Find a counselor through your work, your health provider, or trusted friends, and make an appointment.
- Choose one person that you'd like to forgive—make it something easy—and spend the month reminding yourself that you are letting it go. Then let it go. Hanging on to grudges and slights is stressful and takes away from your quality of life.
- Say "thank you" at least ten times a day for a month. Keep track.
- Take a meditation class. Practice at least three times a week for a month. Notice how you feel.
- Have sex with someone you love. (Even if that is yourself!) Orgasm releases oxytocin, a peptide hormone secreted by your hypothalamus that gives you a feeling of well-being, and is known as "the bonding hormone" because it has the effect of emotional bonding.

- Get a massage. Massage can release toxins you may be holding in your muscles, and can help you relax.

Any of these activities can create a healthy emotional state. Practicing them over a month's time can turn them into lifetime habits that improve your overall emotional well-being.

Screening Checklist

Another part of an effective health maintenance plan is staying on the lookout for possible problems and tending to them in early stages, while they are still treatable.

Getting yearly checkups is a minimum for staying on top of emerging health risks. Your doctor or health care provider will discuss the type of tests that you should undergo every year, based on your family and personal medical histories and your lifestyle. Listed below are some of the components that any annual exam should include:

Annual Exam Checklist		
What?	Who?	How Often?
Human Papilloma	Every woman	Every year with Pap if recent history of STD, or if practicing unsafe sex; every 3 years if Pap and HPV are negative
Pap smear	Every woman	Every 3 years (with negative HPV Screen)
Pelvic and rectal exam	Every woman	Every year
Breast exam	Every woman	Every year by a professional healthcare provider; every month by you
Blood pressure	Every woman	Every year
Cholesterol	Every woman	Every three years if initial test is normal; more often as prescribed
Mammogram	Every woman age forty+	Baseline at forty; every one to two years to age fifty; then every year

Fecal occult blood test	Every woman	Annually after age fifty; after age forty if you have a family history
Electrocardiogram (ECG)	Anyone with two risk factors (family history, heart disease, smoking, diabetes, high blood pressure) high cholesterol	
Bone density	Any woman with risk factors for osteoporosis, every woman age sixty-five and older	Every year
Sigmoidoscopy or colonoscopy	Every woman age 50+	Every five years if findings are normal
Skin cancer check	Every woman	Annually by professional, monthly by you
Blood glucose check	Every woman age 45+	Every three years

These regular screening checks will help you stay on top of your changing body as it approaches and moves through menopause.

Taking a month-by-month approach to your health maintenance plan is a slow, sure way to walk toward a healthier, more comfortable rest of your life. If you don't reach your goal in a given month, put it on the next month's list and give it another shot. After six months, look back and see if you've made enough changes to get you closer to your healthy self. If not, talk to your health care provider about other ways to support your Health Maintenance Plan.

Index

Abdominal fat, 229, 281
ACE inhibitors, 161
Acne, 115
Acupressure, 173
Acupuncture, 22, 89, 130, 172–73
African Americans, 198, 201, 213, 267
AIDS/HIV, 117, 118
Alcohol use, 10, 48, 54, 68, 80, 84, 88, 97, 162, 201, 235, 236, 260, 267
   breast cancer and, 180
   heart disease and, 206
   osteoporosis and, 213, 214, 218
   sexual function and, 116
Alendronate (Fosomax), 220, 221
Alpha hydroxy acids (AHAs), 273–74
Alprazolam, 105, 162
Alzheimer's disease, 77, 78, 143, 167, 241, 254, 256
Amenorrhea, 26, 212
Amitriptyline, 105
Androgens, 5, 66, 139, 142, 145, 273
Anemia, 65, 67, 68
Angina, 192
Anticonvulsants, 213, 219
Antidepressants, 57–58, 86, 104–5, 106, 113, 159–60, 162–63
Antioxidants, 226, 236, 267, 274
Anxiety, 22, 39, 82, 99–100, 105, 162–63, 167, 241
Anxiolytics, 105, 162–63
Arthritis, 8, 32, 72, 74, 83, 113, 248
   osteo-, 173, 231
   rheumatoid, 142
Asians, 198, 213
Aspartame, 88
Asthma, 49
Atherosclerosis, 191, 192, 196, 201

Bellergal, 58
Beta-blockers, 160
Biofeedback, 22, 68, 71, 86, 88, 89, 92, 136, 173–74, 202
Bioflavonoids, 169
Bioidentical hormones, 151–52
Bipolar disorder, 101

Birth control, 117, 123. *See also* Oral contraceptives
Bisphosphonates, 220
Black cohosh, 60–61, 166
Blood clots, 20, 57, 149, 152, 153, 154, 196
Blood sugar/glucose, 5, 68, 90, 105, 141, 168, 202, 256
Body mass index (BMI), 203, 204, 230
Bone density, 142, 145, 168
Bone loss, 20, 22, 49, 73, 161, 241. *See also* Osteoporosis
Bone mineral density (BMD) test, 154, 186, 208, 210–11, 214
Botox, 272
Brain, 103. *See also* Cognitive and neurological changes
   activities for, 256–58
   adaptability of, 80
   age-related changes in, 253–55
   development in later years, 283–84
   exercise and, 241, 255–56
   plasticity of, 287
   shrinkage of, 75, 78–79, 253
Breathing techniques, 55, 61, 107, 173
Buspirone, 105, 162

CA-125, 185
Caffeine, 43, 48, 54, 68, 85, 88, 91, 107, 162, 235–36
Calcitonin, 220, 221
Calcium, 5, 49, 140, 141, 150, 161, 209, 212, 213, 214–17, 218, 235, 270
   recommended intake of, 215, 225
   supplements, 216–17
Calcium channel blockers, 161
Calories, burning, 230, 242
Cancer, 8, 32, 90, 113, 140, 155, 168, 178–85, 231, 239, 244
   breast, 20, 57, 60, 148, 150, 152–53, 154, 157, 160, 166, 171, 172, 176, 179–81, 184, 241
   cervical, 4
   colon/colorectal, 32, 56, 144, 147, 154, 184, 227, 241

endometrial, 20, 42, 56, 57, 64, 142, 148, 171, 181–83, 184
lung, 178–79, 205
ovarian, 171, 172, 183–85, 241
pancreatic, 184
uterine, 152–53, 172
Carlson, Richard, 282
Cataracts, 267–68
Caucasians, 213
Centers for Disease Control and Prevention (CDC), 240, 245
Change and loss, coping with, 281, 282–83
Chasteberry, 168
Chemical peels and dermabrasion, 272
Chemotherapy, 4, 113, 114
Childlessness, cancer risk and, 182, 184
Children, 9, 35
Chocolate, 226
Cholesterol levels, 22, 73, 115, 141, 153, 170, 176, 178, 195–96, 199–200, 206, 231. See also HDL cholesterol; LDL cholesterol
androgens and, 145
diet and, 200, 227
estrogen and, 5
exercise and, 200, 239, 240, 244
menopausal hormone therapy and, 20, 144, 154, 196
nonhormonal medications for, 160–61
Chronic disease, 7–8
Chronic fatigue syndrome, 83
Chunking of information, 261
Citalopram (Prozac; Zoloft; Paxil; Celexa), 105
Clonidine hydrochloride, 57, 159
Coenzyme Q, 255
Coffee, 68. See also Caffeine
Cognitive and neurological changes, 44–46, 75, 77–92. See also Brain; Concentration difficulties; Dizziness; Headaches; Insomnia; Memory; Mental function
Cognitive behavioral therapy, 22, 106, 174
Cohen, Gene, 285
Collagen, 49, 141, 219, 271, 272, 273, 274
Colonoscopy, 32
Computers, working on, 266
Concentration difficulties, 39, 44, 79–80, 167

Confucius, 290
Constipation, 75
Contributing to the world, 285–87
Copper, 267
Coronary artery disease, 191, 192
Coronary microvascular syndrome, 197
Creativity, 289–90
Cues, memory, 261

Dementia, 143, 167, 255. See also Alzheimer's disease
Dendrites, 79, 254, 283–84, 286
Depression, 22, 33, 34, 78, 82, 98, 99, 100–106, 113, 168. See also Antidepressants
causes of, 103
exercise and, 242, 248
major, 101, 103, 104
medical causes of, 104
postpartum, 101, 104
prevalence of, 100–101
symptoms of, 101–2
treatment for, 103–6, 162
Desipramine, 105
DHEA, 168
Diabetes, 7, 32, 49, 72, 168, 186, 201, 231, 267
exercise and, 239, 240, 244, 248
heart disease and, 202–3
Diet, 155, 200, 201–2, 206, 214–17, 223–36, 309–10
after forty, 223–24
avoiding fads, 231–32
breast cancer and, 180
emotional stability and, 107
good habits, 232–34
guidelines for, 234–36
mental function and, 255
nutritional boosts, 225–28
sexual fitness and, 115
weight management and, 229–34
Dietary Supplement Health and Education Act (DSHEA), 165
Diuretics, 160
Dizziness, 89–90
Dong quai, 168
Don't Sweat the Small Stuff (Carlson), 282
Dual energy X-ray absorptiometry (DEXA), 210
Duke Activity Status Index, 197
Dysmenorrhea, 26
Dysthymia, 101

Eating disorders, 213
Eflornithine, 276
Eggs, running out of, 29–30
Elaborative encoding, 260
Embolization, 65, 66
Emotional and psychological changes,
    33–34, 46–49, 93–108. *See also*
    Anxiety; Depression; Mood swings
Endometriosis, 172
Endorphins, 107, 241
Erectile dysfunction, 10, 19, 120
Estradiol, 151
Estriol, 151
Estrogen, 30, 41, 44, 46, 64, 69,
    73, 114, 139, 147, 149, 151, 180,
    184, 195–96, 269, 271
    concentration and, 79
    decline of and health risks, 176
    delivery options, 150
    designer, 152–53, 172, 220–21
    hearing and, 272
    hot flashes and, 52
    memory and, 5, 77–78, 255
    in menopausal hormone therapy, 141–42
    mental function and, 255
    mood swings and, 94, 95
    osteoporosis and, 56, 211–12, 215, 219,
        220–21
    production of, 29
    properties and functions of, 5
    sexual functioning and, 19
    unopposed, 141, 142, 148, 182
    vision and, 266
Estrogen patch, 114, 150
Estrogen therapy (ET), 6–7, 56, 117,
    142–43, 182–83, 196, 229, 255
Estrone, 151
Exercise, 7, 54, 74, 75, 91, 155, 161, 200,
    201–2, 206, 213, 214, 218, 237–52, 310
    aerobic, 244–46
    before bed (avoiding), 85, 242
    breast cancer and, 180–81
    choosing a program, 249
    emotional stability and, 107, 108
    flexibility training, 247–48
    menopause symptom management
        and, 241–43
    mental function and, 255–56
    sexual fitness and, 115, 122
    strength (resistance) training, 218,
        246–47, 248

Eyes/vision, 49, 142, 147, 226, 264–68

Family life, 13, 34–35
Fat, dietary, 235
Fertility, 65
Fiber, 227
Fibroids, uterine, 64–67, 172
Fibromyalgia, 83, 173
Fish, 227, 228, 235
Fluoxetine, 57, 105
Focused ultrasound surgery (FUS), 66
Folates, 255
Follicle-stimulating hormone
    (FSH), 5, 29, 30
Food and Drug Administration
    (FDA), 58, 115, 150, 151, 163,
    165, 167, 220, 221, 226, 228
Friends, 35
Frontal lobes, 78–79, 253, 260–61

Gabapentin, 58, 160
Gardner, Howard, 289
Gingko bilioba, 167
Ginseng root, 168
Glaucoma, 142, 267
Goals, 288–89
Gonadotropin-releasing
    hormone agonists, 66
Green tea, 169, 236
Grief, 283

Hair, 49, 271, 275–76
    body and facial, 115, 145, 273, 275, 276
HDL cholesterol, 73, 153, 154,
    170, 178, 199, 200
Headaches, 45–46, 86–89. *See
    also* Migraine headaches
Health care providers, 125–38
    complementary/alternative care,
        129–31
    finding, 131–33
    traditional, 128–29
Health history, 189–90
Healthy Women's Study, 237
Hearing, 74, 268–69, 272
Heart attacks, 68–69, 100, 177, 191,
    192–93, 196, 197, 201, 205
Heart disease, 7–8, 32, 73–74, 82, 91, 113,
    139–40, 154, 176–78, 191–206, 231, 281
    defined, 191
    diet and, 206, 227–28

exercise and, 206, 239, 240, 244
gender differences in, 197
gum disease and, 270
menopausal hormone therapy and,
    196
risk control, 206
risk factors for, 198–205
symptoms of, 192, 197
Heart palpitations, 31, 39,
    42–43, 45, 68–69
Herbal/botanical treatments,
    59–61, 163–68
Herbalists, 130
Hippocampus, 79, 254, 256, 257, 260
Homeopaths, 130
Hormone replacement therapy
    (HRT), 6–7, 16, 140, 225. *See also*
    Menopausal hormone therapy
Hormones. *See also* specific hormones
    emotions and, 93–94
    fluctuations of, 63–64, 77
    insomnia and, 81–82
    menopause effects on, 5–6, 29
    role of in health, 139
    sexuality and, 113, 114–15
Hot flashes, 31, 39, 51–62, 68,
    82, 92, 95, 153, 173, 174
    the body during, 52–53
    exercise and, 54, 241, 243
    herbal/botanical treatments for,
        59–61, 166, 168
    lessening discomfort of, 22, 54–55
    menopausal hormone therapy and,
        20, 21, 55–57, 142, 146, 147
    mind-body exercises for, 61–62
    nonhormonal medications for, 57–59,
        159–60
    number, length, and intensity of,
        53–54
    percentage of women experiencing,
        20, 41, 51
    phytoestrogens and, 169–70, 227
    range of symptoms, 51–52
    triggers of, 53
Hyperparathyroidism, 212
Hyperplasia, endometrial,
    64, 152, 181, 183
Hypersomnia, 81
Hypertension, 10, 32, 83, 113, 176–77,
    200–202, 204, 231, 235, 266
    exercise and, 201–2, 239, 244

nonhormonal medications for,
    160–61
Hyperventilation, 89, 92
Hypnotics, 86, 163
Hypotension, 90
Hysterectomy, 3, 4, 66–67, 142,
    144, 146–47, 148, 182
Hysteroscopy, 67

Imipramine, 105
Incontinence (urinary), 31,
    39, 43, 69, 70–71, 135
    stress, 43, 69, 70–71, 118, 142, 174
    urge, 43, 69, 70, 142
Insomnia, 22, 39, 45, 48, 80–86, 104,
    163, 167, 168, 241. *See also* Sleep
    medications for, 86, 161–62
    understanding and treating, 82–86
Interpersonal therapy, 106
Isoflavones, 59, 169, 170–72

Kava, 167
Kegel exercise, 71, 118–19
Kidney infections, 188
Kinsey, Alfred, 48
Kliger, Leah, 19

Lasofoxifene, 153
LDL cholesterol, 73, 153, 154, 170,
    178, 196, 199, 200, 227, 240
LEVITY program, 108
Lignans, 169
Lipoic acid, 255
Lithium, 213
Liver disease/dysfunction,
    57, 149, 154, 160, 167
"Living to 100 Life Expectancy
    Calculator," 254
Lungs, changes in, 75
Luteinizing hormone (LH), 29, 52, 166

MacArthur Study of Successful Aging, 281
Macular degeneration, 142,
    147, 226, 266–67
Male menopause (andropause), 9–11
Mammograms, 32, 148
Marriage, 34. *See also* Same-
    sex relationships
Massage, therapeutic, 173
Masters and Johnson, 18, 111
Masturbation, 119, 187

Meaning, finding, 284–85
Meditation, 55, 61, 107, 173, 206, 277
Medroxyprogesterone, 56
Megestrol acetate, 56
Memory, 5, 44–45, 77–79, 167, 253–54,
    255, 256, 259, 283
  methods to enhance, 260–62
Men, 112, 195, 196. *See also* Male menopause
Menarche, 26
Menopausal hormone therapy
    (MHT), 55–57, 74, 91, 106, 129,
    139–55, 180, 196, 219. *See also*
    Hormone replacement therapy
  alternatives to, 22, 157–74
  benefits of, 147–48
  characteristics of users, 146–47
  delivery options, 149–52
  low-dose, 150, 151
  risks of, 148–49
  weighing risks and benefits, 20–21,
    153–55
Menopause. *See also* Perimenopause
  causes of, 29–30
  common wisdom and myths, 17–22
  defined, 1
  finding support for, 23
  heart disease and, 194–97
  induced, 3–4, 143
  in mates, 9–11
  medical impacts of, 159
  medicalization of, 158
  natural, 3
  number of women at or near, 8
  osteoporosis and, 211–12
  timing of, 2–4, 30
Menopause Journal, 29, 154, 299–302
Menorrhea, 26
Menstruation, 25–27. *See also* Periods
Mental function, 253–62. *See also* Brain;
    Cognitive and neurological changes
Methyldopa, 57
Mexican Americans, 198
Midlife crisis, 10, 283
Migraine headaches, 39, 45–46,
    83, 86, 87–88, 92, 149
Minoxidil (Rogaine), 275
Modern Maturity Sexual Survey, 19
Monosodium glutamate (MSG), 88, 107
Mood swings, 34, 39, 46–47, 94–96, 241
  myths about, 19–20
  tracking, 95–96

Multiple sclerosis, 90, 92
Myolysis, 66
Myomectomy, 66

Native Americans, 198
Naturopaths, 129
Nedelman, Deborah, 19
Neurons, 79, 255–56
New England Centenarian Study, 256
Night sweats, 41, 52, 80, 82,
    146, 159–60, 162
Nonhormonal medications, 57–59, 159–63
Non-steroidal anti-inflammatory
    drugs (NSAIDs), 65, 92
North American Menopause
    Society (NAMS), 2, 131–32,
    153, 158, 170, 171, 172–73
Nurse practitioners, 129
Nurses Health Study, 180, 196
Nutritional/dietary supplements, 163–65

Obesity/overweight, 10, 71, 82, 177,
    186, 230–31. *See also* Weight gain
  breast cancer and, 180
  diabetes and, 202
  endometrial cancer and, 182
  heart disease and, 203–4, 206
  hypertension and, 201, 204
  osteoarthritis and, 248
  prevalence of, 73
Obstetrician/gynecologists, 129
Omega-3 fatty acids, 227–28
Ontario Project on Successful Aging, 285
Optimism, 106, 279–80
Oral contraceptives, 65–66, 184.
    See also Birth control
Osteopenia, 186
Osteoporosis, 32, 74, 140, 176,
    185–86, 207–21, 225, 270. *See
    also* Bone density; Bone loss
  characteristics of, 207–8
  diagnosis of, 210–11
  diet and, 214–17
  exercise and, 213, 214, 218, 239, 241,
    245, 248
  fractures caused by, 74, 144, 147, 171,
    185–86, 207, 209, 210, 211,
    214, 219, 220
  menopausal hormone therapy and,
    20, 56, 144, 146, 147, 150,
    152–53, 154, 219

onset of, 208
prevalence of, 207
preventive measures, 217–21
soy and, 170–71
understanding and controlling risks,
    213–14
Otosclerosis, 91
Ovaries, surgical removal of, 3
Ovulation, 25, 29, 30, 63, 64,
    143, 144, 182, 184

Panic attacks, 39, 100, 104, 162
Pap smears, 32, 183
Parathyroid gland, 212, 220
Parents, caring for, 36
Paresthesias, 92
Parkinson's disease, 90, 142, 168
Paroxetine, 57, 105
Perimenopause, 30–36, 37–50
changes during (see Cognitive
    and neurological changes;
    Emotional and psychological
    changes; Physical changes)
defined, 2, 30
health concerns, 30
onset and duration of, 37
sharing feelings about, 12–14
social and family concerns, 34–36
symptoms of, 38–40
Periods, 26–27, 30
heavy, 31, 39, 41–42, 64–67
irregular, 31, 39, 41–42, 63–64, 149,
    213
Perls, Thomas, 254
Pessaries, 71
Phobias, 100
Physical changes, 40–43, 63–75
Phytohormones/estrogens, 22,
    59, 141, 169–73, 227
Pilates, 250
Pituitary gland, 29, 52, 141
Plaque (arterial), 191, 192, 197, 199
Polyps, uterine, 64, 67, 152
Post formal thought, 284
PQRST technique, 261–62
Pregnancy, 60, 166
Premenstrual dysphoric disorder
    (PMDD), 28–29, 105, 162
Premenstrual syndrome (PMS),
    27–29, 47, 56, 79, 81, 101, 104
Presbyopia, 265

Progesterone, 29, 30, 41, 64, 73, 94,
    114, 139, 142, 148, 180, 182
in menopausal hormone therapy,
    143–44
properties and functions of, 5
Progesterone cream, 56, 150
Progestin, 56, 140, 142, 144,
    145, 147, 150, 272
Psychotherapy, 106
Pyelonephritis, 70

Radiation therapy, 4, 113
Radical Acceptance, 287
Radiofrequency treatments, 273
Raloxifene (Evista), 152–53, 220
Red clover, 169, 171–72
Relaxation techniques, 22, 86, 88,
    89, 92, 107, 202, 206, 276–77
Remifem, 166
Reproductive endocrinologists, 129
Rest, 108, 115–16, 276–77
Retinol, 274
Risedronate (Actonel), 220, 221
Roman room technique, 261

Salt/sodium, 91, 107, 206, 235
SAMe, 168
Same-sex relationships, 11, 112
Seasonal Affective Disorder (SAD), 28
Seattle Midlife Women's Health Study, 78
Selective estrogen receptor modulators
    (SERMs), 152–53, 172, 220–21
Selective serotonin reuptake inhibitors
    (SSRIs), 57–58, 105, 162
Selenium, 116, 255
Serotonin, 79, 94, 95
Sertraline, 105
Sex and Aging--Expectations and Reality
    (Masters and Johnson study), 111
Sexuality, 7, 48, 109–23
attitudes toward, 111–13
health maintenance and, 116–20
myths and fears, 18–19, 109–11
orgasm, 111, 113
painful intercourse, 39, 65, 110, 113,
    114
professional counseling and, 119–20,
    121
relationships and, 112–13, 120–21
Sexuality at Midlife and
    Beyond study, 120

Sexually transmitted diseases (STDs), 117
Skin, 49, 271–75
Sleep, 88, 108, 155, 242, 259.
    See also Insomnia
Sleep apnea, 82, 83, 104, 163
Smoking, 43, 71, 75, 85, 97, 116, 155,
    177, 178–79, 201, 204–5, 206,
    213, 214, 218, 266, 267, 274
Soy, 22, 59–60, 141, 169, 170–71, 227, 235
Spotting, 41, 64, 149, 183
Statins, 160, 200
Steroids, 213, 219
Still Sexy After All These Years?
    (Kliger and Nedelman), 19
Stress, 55, 78, 82–83, 96–98,
    115–16, 239, 276, 277
    exercise and, 256
    heart disease and, 206
    managing, 97, 99, 281–82
    at work, 98
Stress hormones, 80, 281
Stroke, 90, 177, 191, 192, 196, 197,
    201, 202, 227, 231, 270
Sugar, 43, 48, 107, 270

Tai chi, 107, 251, 277
Tamoxifen (Nolvadex), 152
Teeth and gums, 269–71
Testosterone therapy, 10, 115, 142, 180
Thyroid disorders, 68, 91, 104, 276
Thyroid hormone replacement, 213, 219
Tingling/burning sensations, 92
Tinnitus, 91–92
Trichomoniasis, 186
Tricyclic antidepressants, 86, 105
Triglycerides, 154, 170, 196, 199, 200
20/20/20 rule, 266

Urinary tract infections (UTIs),
    43, 69, 70, 186, 187–88

Vaginal atrophy, 110, 114, 153, 176, 187
Vaginal dryness, 7, 20, 21, 39, 110, 113,
    117, 145, 146, 147, 168, 171, 187
Vaginal health, 117–18, 141, 142
Vaginitis, 186–87
Vegetarianism, 216
Venlafaxine, 57
Vestibular disorders, 90
Visualization, 55, 61, 62
Vitamins, 225–26

A, 226, 267, 274
B12, 80
C, 226, 267, 274
D, 49, 140, 150, 161, 215–16, 217, 218,
    226
E, 60, 116, 226, 255, 267, 274
    recommended daily intake, 224
    supplements, 116, 216–17, 229

Walking, 218, 250, 252
Warfarin (Coumadin), 168
Water intake, 54, 229, 270, 274, 275
Weight gain, 31, 32, 39, 43, 49,
    71–73, 83, 203–4, 225. *See
    also* Obesity/overweight
    genetic factors in, 72–73
    managing, 229–34
    myths about, 19–21
Wisdom, 254
Women's Health Initiative (WHI)
    study, 6, 21, 139–41, 143, 144, 148,
    150, 151, 152, 180, 196, 255
Women's health nurse
    practitioners (WHNPs), 129
Wong, Paul T. P., 285

Yeast infections, 186–87
Yoga, 55, 61, 62, 107, 173, 250, 277

Zinc, 116, 267